Juvenile Myoclonic Epilepsy: The Janz Syndrome

Juvenile Myoclonic Epilepsy:
The Janz Syndrome

Edited by

BETTINA SCHMITZ and THOMAS SANDER

Charité Medical Faculty, Virchow Campus,
Humboldt University, Berlin, Germany

WRIGHTSON BIOMEDICAL PUBLISHING LTD
Petersfield, UK and Philadelphia, USA

Editorial Office:

Wrightson Biomedical Publishing Ltd
Ash Barn House, Winchester Road, Stroud,
Petersfield, Hampshire GU32 3PN, UK
Telephone: 44 (0)1730 265647
Fax: 44 (0)1730 260368

British Library Cataloguing in Publication Data
Juvenile myoclonic epilepsy : the Janz syndrome
   1. Spasms, Infantile 2. Myoclonus – genetic aspects
   I. Schmitz, Bettina II. Sander, Thomas
   618.9'2'853

Library of Congress Cataloging in Publication Data
Juvenile myoclonic epilepsy : the Janz syndrome/edited by
Bettins Schmitz and Thomas Sander
    p.; cm.
   Includes bibliographical references and index.
   ISBN 1-871816-42-4 (hardcover)
   1. Myoclonus. 2. Epilepsy in adolescence. I. Schmitz, Bettina, 1960–.
   II.Sander, Thomas, 1956–
   [DNLM: 1. Epilepsy, Myoclonic–Adolescence. WL 385 J97 2000]
   RJ496.E6 J885 2000
   616.8'53'00835–dc21   99-058336

ISBN 1 871816 42 4

Composition by Scribe Design, Gillingham, Kent
Printed in Great Britain by Biddles Ltd, Guildford

Contents

Contributors vii

Preface ix

1 Dieter Janz and the Janz Syndrome: Gestalt Perception and
   Analysis
   Peter Wolf 1

2 Juvenile Myoclonic Epilepsy: The European History
   Dieter Scheffner 5

3 Juvenile Myoclonic Epilepsy Today: Current Definition and Limits
   Pierre Genton, Philippe Gélisse and Pierre Thomas 11

4 Juvenile Myoclonic Epilepsy: A Syndrome Challenging Syndromic
   Concepts?
   Peter Wolf and Thomas Mayer 33

5 The EEG in Juvenile Myoclonic Epilepsy
   Stephan Waltz 41

6 Pathophysiology of Myoclonus in Janz Syndrome
   G. Avanzini, S. Binelli, S. Franceschetti, F. Panzica and A. Pozzi .. 57

7 Juvenile Myoclonic Epilepsy with Praxis-Induced Seizures
   Yushi Inoue and Hidemoto Kubota 73

8 Structural Changes in Juvenile Myoclonic Epilepsy: Evidence from
   Quantitative MRI
   Friedrich G. Woermann and John S. Duncan 83

9 Positron Emission Tomography in Idiopathic Generalized Epilepsy:
   Imaging Beyond Structure
   Matthias J. Koepp and John S. Duncan 91

10 Cognitive and Personality Profiles in Patients with Juvenile
   Myoclonic Epilepsy
   Michael Trimble 101

v

11 Response to Antiepileptic Drugs and the Rate of Relapse after
    Discontinuation in Juvenile Myoclonic Epilepsy
    Dieter Schmidt 111

12 Maternal Use of Valproate during Pregnancy: Risk of Major
    Malformations and Brain Disorders
    Sabine Koch, Karl Titze, Silvia Treuter, Michael Schröder,
    Ralf B. Zimmermann, Hans-Christoph Steinhausen, Heinz Nau,
    Ulrike Lehmkuhl and Hellgard Rauh 121

13 Clinical Genetics in Subtypes of Idiopathic Generalized Epilepsies
    Bettina Schmitz, Ulrike Sailer, Thomas Sander, Gerhard Bauer and
    Dieter Janz 129

14 The Search for Epilepsy Genes in Juvenile Myoclonic Epilepsy:
    Discoveries Along the Way
    Antonio V. Delgardo-Escueta, Maria E. Alonso, Marco T. Medina,
    Manyee N. Gee and G.C.Y. Fong 145

15 Progress in Mapping the Gene for Juvenile Myoclonic Epilepsy
    (*EJM1*) within the Chromosomal Region 6p21.3
    Thomas Sander, Birgit Bockenkamp, Andreas Ziegler and
    Dieter Janz 173

16 The Major Susceptibility Locus for Juvenile Myoclonic Epilepsy on
    Chromosome 15q
    Louise Bate, Magali Williamson and Mark Gardiner 181

17 Quo Vadis?
    Dieter Janz 197

Index 201

Contributors

Maria E. Alonso, *National Institute of Neurology and Neurosurgery, Mexico City, Mexico*

G. Avanzini, *Department of Neurophysiology, 'C. Besta' National Neurological Institute, 20133 Milan, Italy*

Louise Bate, *Department of Paediatrics, University College London, Rayne Institute, University Street, London WC1E 6JJ, UK*

Gerhard Bauer, *Department of Neurology, University Hospital, Innsbruck, Austria*

S. Binelli, *Department of Neurophysiology, 'C. Besta' National Neurological Institute, 20133 Milan, Italy*

Birgit Bockenkamp, *Department of Neurology and Institute for Immunogenetics, Charité Medical Faculty, Virchow Campus, Humboldt University, 13353 Berlin, Germany*

Antonio V. Delgado-Escueta, *California Comprehensive Epilepsy Program, UCLA School of Medicine and West Los Angeles DVA Medical Center, 11301 Wilshire Boulevard, West Los Angeles, CA 90073, USA*

John S. Duncan, *Institute of Neurology, National Hospital for Neurology and Neurosurgery, Queen Square, London WC1N 3BG, UK*

G.C.Y. Fong, *California Comprehensive Epilepsy Program, UCLA School of Medicine and West Los Angeles DVA Medical Center, 11301 Wilshire Boulevard, West Los Angeles, CA 90073, USA*

S. Franceschetti, *Department of Neurophysiology, 'C. Besta' National Neurological Institute, 20133 Milan, Italy*

Mark Gardiner, *Department of Paediatrics, University College London, Rayne Institute, University Street, London WC1E 6JJ, UK*

Manyee N. Gee, *California Comprehensive Epilepsy Program, UCLA School of Medicine and West Los Angeles DVA Medical Center, 11301 Wilshire Boulevard, West Los Angeles, CA 90073, USA*

Philippe Gélisse, *Centre Saint Paul, 13258 Marseille 09, France*

Pierre Genton, *Centre Saint Paul, 13258 Marseille 09, France*

Yushi Inoue, *National Epilepsy Centre, Shizuoka Higashi Hospital, Urushiyama 886, Shizuoka 420-8688, Japan*

Dieter Janz, *Epilepsy Research Group, Charité Medical Faculty, Virchow Campus, Humboldt University, 13353 Berlin, Germany*

Sabine Koch *Rehabilitationsklinik für Kinder und Jugendliche, Kartzow-Beelitz in Beelitz-Heilstätten, Germany*

Matthias J. Koepp, *Institute of Neurology, National Hospital for Neurology and Neurosurgery, Queen Square, London WC1N 3BG, UK*

Hidemoto Kubota, *National Epilepsy Centre, Shizuoka Higashi Hospital, Urushiyama 886, Shizuoka 420-8688, Japan*

Ulrike Lehmkuhl, *Department of Child and Adolescent Psychiatry, Psychosomatic Medicine and Psychotherapy, Charité Medical Faculty, Virchow Campus, Humboldt University, 13353 Berlin, Germany*

Thomas Mayer, *Epilepsie-Zenbrum Bethel, 33617 Bielefeld, Germany*

Marco T. Medina, *California Comprehensive Epilepsy Program, UCLA School of Medicine and West Los Angeles DVA Medical Center, 11301 Wilshire Boulevard, West Los Angeles, CA 90073, USA*

Heinz Nau, *Department of Food Toxicology, College of Veterinary Medicine, Hannover, Germany*

F. Panzica, *Department of Neurophysiology, 'C. Besta' National Neurological Institute, 20133 Milan, Italy*

A. Pozzi, *Department of Neurophysiology, 'C. Besta' National Neurological Institute, 20133 Milan, Italy*

Hellgard Rauh, *Institute for Psychology, University of Potsdam, Germany*

Ulrike Sailer, *Department of Neurology, University Hospital, Innsbruck, Austria*

Thomas Sander, *Epilepsy Genetics Group, Charité Medical Faculty, Virchow Campus, Humboldt University, 13353 Berlin, Germany*

Dieter Scheffner, *Charité Medical Faculty, Virchow Campus, Humboldt University, 13353 Berlin, Germany*

Dieter Schmidt, *Epilepsy Research Group, Berlin, Germany*

Bettina Schmitz, *Department of Neurology, Charité Medical Faculty, Virchow Campus, Humboldt University, 13353 Berlin, Germany*

Michael Schröder, *Department of Neurology, Charité Medical Faculty, Virchow Campus, Humboldt University, 13353 Berlin, Germany*

Hans-Christoph Steinhausen, *Department of Child and Adolescent Psychiatry, University of Zurich, Switzerland*

Pierre Thomas, *Department of Neurology, Hôpital Pasteur, Nice, France*

Karl Titze, *Department of Child and Adolescent Psychiatry, Psychosomatic Medicine and Psychotherapy, Charité Medical Faculty, Virchow Campus, Humboldt University, 13353 Berlin, Germany*

Silvia Treuter, *Department of Child and Adolescent Psychiatry, Psychosomatic Medicine and Psychotherapy, Charité Medical Faculty, Virchow Campus, Humboldt University, 13353 Berlin, Germany*

Michael Trimble, *Institute of Neurology, National Hospital for Neurology and Neurosurgery, Queen Square, London WC1N 3BG, UK*

Stephan Waltz, *Neuropaediatric Department, University of Kiel, 24105 Kiel, Germany*

Magali Williamson, *Department of Pediatrics, University College London, Rayne Institute, University Street, London WC1E 6JJ, UK*

Peter Wolf, *Epilepsie-Zentrum Bethel, 33617 Bielefeld, Germany*

Friedrich G. Woermann, *The MRI Unit, National Society of Epilepsy, Chalfont St Peter, Gerrards Cross, Buckinghamshire SL9 0RJ, UK*

Andreas Ziegler, *Department of Neurology and Institute for Immunogenetics, Charité Medical Faculty, Virchow Campus, Humboldt University, 13353 Berlin, Germany*

Ralf B. Zimmermann, *Department of Neurology, Charité Medical Faculty, Virchow Campus, Humboldt University, 13353 Berlin, Germany*

Preface

Why publish an epilepsy book at the beginning of the 21st Century on a syndrome which has been well defined for some forty years? At first sight juvenile myoclonic epilepsy, or JME, appears to be a 'simple' epilepsy syndrome, easy to recognize by the experienced neurologist and easy to control in most cases. However, we believe that this syndrome still has exciting secrets, some of which, such as specific reflex mechanisms, have only recently been discovered.

Following a decade when epileptology seemed to be reduced to investigating focal epilepsies and surgical treatment, there is now growing interest in the idiopathic generalized epilepsies, in part due to progress in molecular biology and clinical research.

Genetic studies of juvenile myoclonic epilepsy provide an ideal model for investigating and understanding epileptogenesis on a molecular level. The development of sensitive imaging techniques has allowed the identification of subtle functional and morphological lesions, which has rekindled conceptual discussions about the distinction between idiopathic vebrsus symptomatic epilepsies, and generalized versus focal epilepsy syndromes.

The early observation by Dieter Janz that the syndrome is characterized not only by specific types of seizures but also by a specific behavioural profile, including a typical sleep and wake pattern in relationship to seizures, has recently aroused further interest amongst psychiatrists, neuropsychologists and electrophysiologists. These, and several other topics, form the basis of this monograph.

The book itself celebrates the 25th anniversary of the Chair of Neurology at the former Klinikum Charlottenburg which was first held by Dieter Janz. All the contributing authors have been involved in cooperative research with Dieter Janz and most have spent some time working in or visiting his department at Charlottenburg, or in the succeeding Department of Neurology at the Charité.

An interest in JME is common to all pupils of Dieter Janz and many of them have contributed to a further understanding of this 'simple' syndrome.

We hope that this book will help spread enthusiasm for epileptology generally; we recognize juvenile myoclonic epilepsy as an ambassador for that subject.

THE EDITORS

Juvenile Myoclonic Epilepsy: The Janz Syndrome
Edited by Bettina Schmitz and Thomas Sander
© 2000 Wrightson Biomedical Publishing Ltd

1

Dieter Janz and the Janz Syndrome: Gestalt Perception and Analysis

PETER WOLF

Epilepsie-Zentrum Bethel, Bielefeld, Germany

When we talk today about juvenile myoclonic epilepsy we think of a characteristic type of myoclonic seizure; we think perhaps of some problems of genetic analysis; we think as clinicians of valproate (VPA); and we certainly think of the poly spike-wave (PSW) pattern which we like to see on the electroencephalogram (EEG) when we want to have this diagnosis confirmed.

Many are astonished to hear that the EEG had only a minor role in the description of Janz syndrome in the mid-1950s because at that time electroencephalography was still a new technique, the importance of which remained to be clearly defined. Impulsive petit mal – as Janz proposed to call this epileptic disorder – was conceived as a clinical syndrome.

For many generations, patients had been telling their doctors about the jerks which sometimes could precede their generalized tonic-clonic (GTC) seizures. Not all patients did this because few found it important, and even fewer would volunteer the information that these jerks sometimes could occur alone without being followed by a grand mal (GM) seizure. Generations of doctors had heard about this trait. Why was Dieter Janz the first to connect it with others, and to ask whether there were any typical conditions under which these jerks occured?

It would seem that four preconditions had to be fulfilled. First, he understood that it is the patients who tell us the most important things about epilepsy, and that it is worth our while to listen carefully to them; secondly, he understood that patients will not always spontaneously give all the information they have: it must be systematically elicited; thirdly, like Jackson with respect to focal epilepsies, Janz must have felt that it is not the study of the maximal symptoms which improves our understanding of epilepsy but, rather, the study of minimal symptoms at the onset of seizures. But, lastly, he had the ability to recognize a certain gestalt which could be found in the reports of some patients. Because, without such a holistic perception of an entire form, the description of the syndrome would certainly not have included such features as physical constitution, personality traits, and the social prognosis.

However, in addition to these, the original description pays attention to features such as the age of onset, precipitating mechanisms of seizures, their relation to the circadian cycle, and even to seemingly remote features such as findings of skull X-rays or such aspects as, in the GM seizures that may follow the jerks, a deeper cyanosis than usual. This illustrates that, even if the main presenting features of the syndrome may have been perceived as a general outline, Dieter Janz and his co-worker Walter Christian soon became aware that this was not enough and that many details had to be considered to complete the picture of the syndrome.

It is the privilege of a young man of genius to have a hitherto unnoticed gestalt revealed to him and to describe it. An artist could have stopped here. In science, however, gestalt perceptions give us ideas, hypotheses, which then need to be investigated. In the original paper, Janz and Christian (1957) used what they called the *Bewegungsmotiv*, i.e. the motor pattern of the typical jerks in their attempt to reach a deeper understanding of the syndrome. They compared the pattern in juvenile myoclonic epilepsy (JME) with that of West syndrome, and with the retroversive movement typical for pyknoleptic absences. They noted that all three patterns develop in the sagittal body axis, and affect the static functions of the body. The different movement directions led them to the terminological conclusion of calling these patterns 'propulsive' (West), 'retropulsive' (pyknolepsy) and 'impulsive' – the latter also a tribute to nineteenth-century French author Herpin (1867) who had called the myocloni *sécousses* or *impulsions*.

In their analysis of the semiology of the disorder, Janz and Christian (1957) compared the motor pattern in this syndrome with patterns seen in other neurological conditions, such as decerebration, and came to the conclusion that the pattern must be generated in the mesencephalon. Epileptological research has not generally followed this line of gestalt analysis but that did not prevent Dieter Janz from focusing his interest on 'impulsive petit mal'.

It took many years before others also began to understand and be aware of this syndrome. It became fully recognized when the International League Against Epilepsy included it in its Proposal for a Classification of Epilepsies and Epileptic Syndromes (Commission on Classification and Terminology of the ILAE, 1985). At that time, however, Dieter Janz was already deeply involved in the study of the genetics of epilepsy and, as good luck would have it, JME soon figured prominently in this research. A new line of analytic approach to the syndrome was opened to which many authors have started to contribute. One result of this is that it is necessary to go back to the clinical syndrome to take a closer analytic look at some details of the phenotype. This volume is mostly concerned with these recent developments.

REFERENCES

Commission on Classification and Terminology of the International League Against Epilepsy (1985). Proposal for classification of epilepsies and epileptic syndromes. *Epilepsia* **26**, 268–278.
Herpin, Th. (1867). *Des Accès Incomplets d'Épilepsie*. Baillière, Paris.
Janz, D. and Christian, W. (1957). Impulsiv-Petit Mal. *J Neurol* **176**, 346–386.

Juvenile Myoclonic Epilepsy: The Janz Syndrome
Edited by Bettina Schmitz and Thomas Sander
© 2000 Wrightson Biomedical Publishing Ltd

2

Juvenile Myoclonic Epilepsy: The European History

DIETER SCHEFFNER

Charité Medical Faculty, Virchow Campus, Humboldt University, Berlin, Germany

The celebration of 25 years of epileptology in Berlin in 1998 provided a good opportunity to focus on juvenile myoclonic epilepsy (JME) and on Dieter Janz, who first recognized this type of idiopathic generalized epilepsy (IGE) of adolescence in 1955 and published on it in full detail together with W. Christian in 1957 (Janz and Christian, 1957, 1994).

Before presenting a short overview on the European history of this type of epilepsy, it is first necessary to illustrate the path that was travelled between recognizing the signs and symptoms, and suspecting a distinct nosology of which the signs might be indicative, to ultimately establishing a correspondence at the molecular level.

'There are epileptic equivalents that look like a sudden contraction, caused by intense fright.' This is the first sentence in the first detailed publication on this topic by Janz and Christian in 1957 which noted a particular type of contraction under certain conditions, which might become meaningful for attributing similar observations to a specific entity.

Tracing the history of JME remains confusing, although Janz himself pursued the trait precisely back. Following his footsteps, however, does not imply merely collecting signs and facts from various observations, but rather trying to find out their meaning and significance. Janz tried to put together seizure elements, impulsions, and conditions of their appearance in a framework in order to understand the underlying pathophysiology. Thus in 1957 he stated: 'From the permanent comparison between symptoms, one can learn to read them as syllables of language of an organ – not unlike the meaning of foreign characters. Then, even if the experimental basis is still missing, one will admit that the performance of the maintenance of body position represents the physiological basis that is affected in different ways, in the seizures of the petit mal triad.' Even bearing in mind the genetic explanation for this type of epilepsy, his statement meant that both the pathological process of the seizure and the biological performance act on the same neurophysiological level (Janz and Christian, 1957, 1994).

Herpin (1867) was the first to name and precisely describe the previously known clinical phenomenon of '... a jerk, which runs through the entire body like an electric current'. He called it a *secousse*, and considered it 'a variety of (seizure)-prelude'. These jerks were also called commotions or impulsions and labelled by other authors prodromes, auras or aborted seizures (see Janz and Christian, 1994).

A constant relation between the myoclonic jerk described by Herpin (1867) and epilepsy was first acknowledged about 30 years after Herpin. In 1899 Dide published *La Myoclonie dans l'Épilepsie* while Rabot in his thesis (1899) attributed it nosologically, indicated by the topic 'La Myoclonie Épileptique'. He also differentiated it as 'petit mal moteur' as distinct from 'petit mal intellectuel'.

Here we will deal briefly with a diversion in relation to JME which has become a long-standing source of confusion and debate (Gastaut *et al.*, 1974). It started with the description of paramyoclonus multiplex by Friedreich (1881). From the different publications following his paper, Unverricht (1891) 'crystallized a specific condition', later called progressive familiar myoclonus, obviously different – and this alone is important for us – from the condition described by Herpin while he and others (Clark and Prout, 1902) considered epileptic fits, occurring in progressive familiar myoclonus epilepsy, a complication of this condition.

Lundborg (1903) clearly differentiated progressive familiar myoclonus epilepsy from intermittent sporadic myoclonus epilepsy of Rabot´s type which he considered close to 'essential' (idiopathic) epilepsy.

About 90 years after Herpin's publication and 60 years after Rabot, the papers by Janz (1955) and Janz and Christian (1957) were eliciting much discussion among German-speaking epileptologists but seemed not to have been appreciated outside Germany. Similarly, Castells and Mendilaharsu's paper from Argentina (1958) dealing with JME did not seem to exert much influence among English-speaking neurologists.

Although the term myoclonia may be considered tautologous and the term myoclonic jerk likewise redundant (Lennox, 1960), myoclonus/myoclonic became widely used for any type of jerking (Lecasble, 1958). It is even applied these days to all epileptic diseases of infancy and early childhood that begin with involuntary arrhythmic jerks, irrespective of their pathogenetic and prognostic differences (Janz *et al.*, 1997; Janz and Durner, 1997).

Coming back to Europe, and especially to Germany, the term 'impulsive petit mal (PM)' was preferred. Since 1959 in the German textbook on seizures in childhood by Bamberger and Matthes, impulsive PM constitutes the PM triad together with propulsive PM (West syndrome), and retropulsive PM (Friedmann syndrome).

Kruse (1968) and also Christian (1968) come back to the concept of a PM quartet, reviving a suggestion by Lennox and Davis (1950) in which impulsive PM constitutes the fourth type of age-dependent PM syndrome. Since then, impulsive PM has been included in every textbook on epilepsy, paediatrics or neurology published in the German language.

It was not until 1972/73 that Janz introduced impulsive PM officially to an international forum, the Colloque de Marseille, which in 1972 exceptionally was held in Venice; this took place nearly 20 years after he had first described it. Janz complained that his description of the disease had found no echo outside German-speaking countries. He could not believe that impulsive PM could be a purely teutonic variety of epilepsy. Gastaut replied that he already had described the same syndrome previously, however, he had not considered it nosologically an entity.

The theory Janz presented in Venice and which he had already noted in his first publication was not merely the description of a single syndrome which he differentiated from many others. He was the first to present a well-delineated nosological entity. The clinical picture of this age-dependent syndrome is rooted in the idiopathic generalized epilepsies: pyknoleptic childhood absences; juvenile absence epilepsy; juvenile myoclonic epilepsy; and grand mal epilepsy on awakening.

Each of this quartet may present alone, more often combined with one or two of the others, or one variant of the quartet may be followed by another. They are linked by their relation to the sleep-wake cycle to which Janz's research was devoted, even before he published on impulsive PM. He suggested a basic disturbance in the ability to control sleep and waking in an optimal way.

The occurrence of major and minor seizures is very much influenced by external stimuli. Patients share particular personal and behavioural characteristics (suggestibility, inability to resist temptation) which permit one to exert a therapeutic influence besides drug therapy (Janz, 1973; Leder, 1969; Lund et al., 1976; Gershengorn et al., 1997). The proper role of the suggested frontal lobe dysfunction and microdysgenesis as a common endogenous origin of idiopathic generalized epilepsies (IGEs) beginning in childhood and adolescence has yet to be confirmed by further investigations.

The increased family incidence, the frequent clinical concordance and the results of twin studies link the members of IGE, while EEG studies claim an independent existence within the framework of generalized epilepsies (Tsuboi and Christian, 1973). While the different phenotypes of the quartet can be explained easily it may become more difficult to understand the diversity from the genotypic differentiation.

Thirty years after being described by Janz and Christian, this epileptic entity was rediscovered in the USA and made familiar to the English-speaking world by Asconapé and Penry (1984) and by Delgado-Escueta and Enrile-Bacsal (1984).

REFERENCES

Asconapé, J. and Penry, J.K. (1984). Some clinical and EEG aspects of benign juvenile myoclonic epilepsy. *Epilepsia* **25**, 108–114.

Bamberger, P. and Matthes, A. (1959). *Anfälle im Kindesalter.* Karger, Basel.

Castells, C. and Mendilaharsu, C. (1958). La epilepsia mioclonica bilateral y consciente. *Acta Neurol Lat Am* **4**, 23–48.

Christian, W. (1968). *Klinische Elektroenzephalographie.* Thieme, Stuttgart.

Clark, L.P. and Prout, T.P. (1902). The nature and pathology of myoclonus epilepsy. *Am J Insanity* **59**, 185–223.

Delgado-Escueta, A.V. and Enrile-Bacsal, F. (1984). Juvenile myoclonic epilepsy of Janz. *Neurology* **34**, 285–294.

Dide, M. (1899). *La Myoclonie dans l'Épilepsie.* Paris (cited in Lundborg, H. (1903)). *Die Progressive Myoklonusepilepsie (Unverrichts Myoklonie).* Almquist & Wiksell, Upsala, Sweden.

Friedreich, N. (1881). Neuropathologische Beobachtungen: Paramyoclonus multiplex. *Virchows Arch Pathol Anat* **86**, 421–434.

Gastaut, H., Broughton, R., Roger, J. and Tassinari, C.A. (1974). Generalized convulsive seizures without local onset. In: Vinken, P.J. and Bruyn, G.W. (Eds), *Handbook of Clinical Neurology, Vol 15: The Epilepsies.* Elsevier, Amsterdam, pp. 107–129.

Gershengorn, J., Devinsky, O., Brown, E., Perrine, K., Vasquez, B. and Luciano, D. Frontal functions in juvenile myoclonic epilepsy. Cited in Janz, D. and Durner, M. (1997). Juvenile myoclonic epilepsy. In: Engel J. Jr. and Pedley, T.A. (Eds), *Epilepsy: A Comprehensive Textbook.* Chapter 228, Lippincott-Raven, Philadelphia, PA, pp. 2389–2400.

Herpin, Th. (1867). *Des Accès Incomplets d'Épilepsie.* Baillière, Paris.

Janz, D. (1955). Die klinische Stellung der Pyknolepsie, *Dtsch Med Wochenschr* **80**, 1392–1400.

Janz, D. (1973). The natural history of primary generalized epilepsies with sporadic myoclonias of the 'Impulsive petit mal' type. In: Lugaresi, E., Pazzaglia, P. and Tassinari, C.A. (Eds), *Evolution and Prognosis of Epilepsies.* Gaggi, Bologna, pp. 55–61.

Janz, D. and Christian, W.(1957). *Impulsiv-Petit mal, Dtsch Z. Nervenheilk* **176**, 348–386.

Janz, D. and Christian, W. (1994). Impulsive petit mal. In: Malafosse, A., Genton, P., Hirsch, E., Marescaux, C., Broglin, D. and Bernasconi, R. (Eds), *Idiopathic Generalized Epilepsies: Clinical, Experimental and Genetic Aspects.* John Libbey, London, pp. 229–251.

Janz, D. and Durner, M. (1997). Juvenile myoclonic epilepsy. In: Engel J. Jr. and Pedley, T.A. (Eds), *Epilepsy: A Comprehensive Textbook.* Lippincott-Raven, Philadelphia, PA, pp. 2389–2400.

Janz, D., Inoue, Y. and Seino, M. (1997). Myoclonic seizures. In: Engel J. Jr. and Pedley, T.A. (Eds), *Epilepsy: A Comprehensive Textbook.* Lippincott-Raven, Philadelphia, PA, pp. 591–603.

Kruse, R. (1968). *Das myoklonisch-astatische Petit Mal.* Springer, Heidelberg.

Lecasble, R. (1958). Les myoclonies épileptiques. In: Alajouanine, Th. (Ed.), *Bases Physiologiques et Aspects Cloniques de l'Épilepsie*. Masson, Paris.

Leder, A. (1969). Zur Psychopathologie der Schlaf- und Aufwachepilepsie (Eine psychodiagnostische Untersuchung). *Nervenarzt* **38**, 434–442.

Lennox, W.G. (1960). *Epilepsy and Related Disorders*, Little, Brown, Boston, MD, pp. 122–143.

Lennox, W.G. and Davis, J.P. (1950). Clinical correlates of the fast and slow spike-wave electroencephalogram. *Pediatrics* **5**, 626.

Lund, M., Reintoft, N.M. and Simonsen, N. (1976). Eine kontrollierte soziologische und psychologische Untersuchung von Patienten mit juveniler myoklonischer Epilepsie. *Nervenarzt* **47**, 708–712.

Lundborg, H.B. (1903). *Die progressive Myoklonus Epilepsie (Unverricht's Myoklonie)*. Almquist and Wiksell, Upsala, Sweden.

Rabot, L. (1899). *La myoclonie épileptique* [Thesis]. Paris.

Tsuboi, T. and Christian, W. (1973). On the genetics of the primary generalized epilepsy with sporadic myoclonias of impulsive petit mal type. *Humangenetik* **19**, 155–182.

Unverricht, H.B. (1891). *Die Myoclonie*, Franz Deuticke, Leipzig-Wien.

Juvenile Myoclonic Epilepsy: The Janz Syndrome
Edited by Bettina Schmitz and Thomas Sander
© 2000 Wrightson Biomedical Publishing Ltd

3

Juvenile Myoclonic Epilepsy Today: Current Definition and Limits

PIERRE GENTON*, PHILIPPE GÉLISSE* and PIERRE THOMAS†

Centre Saint Paul, Marseille, and †Department of Neurology, Hôpital Pasteur, Nice, France

INTRODUCTION

One may wonder whether it is still necessary to define juvenile myoclonic epilepsy (JME), a fairly common epileptic syndrome that was recognized more than a century ago and described in detail by Janz and Christian in 1957. It appears, however, that JME remains underdiagnosed at the end of the 20th century, although progress has been made in recent years. Our recent experience may illustrate this point: when we studied retrospectively the electroencephalographic characteristics of JME in 56 consecutive recently diagnosed patients (Genton *et al.*, 1995), we found that none of these had been referred to our specialized epilepsy centre with the diagnosis of JME. In the past five years, however, referring neurologists have suspected increasingly the correct diagnosis, which is proposed prior to referral in nearly half of the cases.

A clear-cut definition of JME has been proposed (Commission on Classification and Terminology of the ILAE, 1989) and accepted by clinicians but geneticists have not had it very easy. It has become clear that identifying the genomic anomaly associated with the disease is very difficult. It has been found that family studies proved a high degree of heterogeneity, with many variations of the phenotype (clinical and electroencephalographic (EEG)) present either between individuals, or within multiplex families. In this chapter we shall however restrict ourselves to the clinical picture, and present here the relevant clinical features found in patients with JME; the EEG characteristics and the genetic context are discussed elsewhere in this volume.

Our recent experience is based on the retrospective study of 170 consecutive JME cases diagnosed in two epilepsy centres (Centre Saint Paul, Marseille, and

Clinique Neurologique, Nice) over the past 15 years: the main clinical characteristics of this patient population are reported in Table 1. The study is also based on many recent reviews of JME (Delgado-Escueta and Enrile-Bacsal, 1984; Asconapé and Penry, 1984; Wolf, 1985; Dinner *et al.*, 1987; Salas-Puig *et al.*, 1990; Janz, 1991; Wolf, 1992a; Serratosa and Delgado-Escueta, 1993; Grünewald and Panayiotopoulos, 1993; Genton *et al.*, 1994; Janz and Durner, 1998). These data and the extensive experience of other authors make it possible to propose an accurate description of JME as it exists in our patients today.

This chapter delineates JME in relation to other conditions, mostly other types of idiopathic generalized epilepsies (IGE). Among the many questions that remain open, one may guide the process of definition: Is JME an epileptic syndrome (i. e. a constellation of symptoms with various aetiologies) or a true epileptic disease? From a strictly clinical point of view, the answer to that question is not easy.

JME: THE DEFINITIONS

The 1989 International Classification of Epilepsies and Related Syndromes (Commission on Classification and Terminology of the ILAE, 1989) gives a fairly precise definition of JME:

Juvenile myoclonic epilepsy appears around puberty and is characterized by seizures with bilateral, single or repetitive, arrhythmic, irregular myoclonic jerks, predominantly in the arms. Jerks may cause some patients to fall suddenly. No disturbance of consciousness is noticeable. The disorder may be inherited, and sex distribution is equal. Often, there are generalized tonic-clonic seizures and, less often, infrequent absences. The seizures usually occur shortly after awakening and are often precipitated by sleep deprivation. Interictal and ictal EEGs have rapid, generalized, often irregular spike-waves and polyspike-waves; there is no close phase correlation between EEG spikes and jerks. Frequently, the patients are photosensitive. Response to appropriate drugs is good.

This definition of JME remains unchallenged and accurate. It was based on sound clinical observation, and includes the electroclinical correlations. The idiopathic generalized epilepsies, the larger group of epilepsies that includes JME, has been defined in the following way in the same text (Commission on Classification and Terminology of the ILAE, 1989):

Idiopathic generalized epilepsies are forms of generalized epilepsies in which all seizures are initially generalized, with an EEG expression that is a generalized, synchronous, symmetrical discharge. The patient usually has a normal interictal state, without neurologic or neuroradiologic signs. In general, interictal EEGs show normal background activity and generalized discharges, such as spikes, polyspike, spike-wave and polyspike-waves (≥ 3 Hz). The discharges are increased by slow sleep. The various syndromes of idiopathic generalized epilepsies vary mainly in age of onset.

Table 1. Main characteristics of our population (MJ, myoclonic jerks; GTCS, generalized tonic-clonic seizures; TA, typical absences).

Age/duration (years)	Mean ± SD	range	
Age on Jan. 1, 1999	32.4 ± 10.4	11.7 – 70.7	
Age at first referral	24.4 ± 9.5	11 – 63.9	
Duration of epilepsy at first referral	9.8 ± 9.5	0 – 49	
Diagnostic delay (n = 137)	7.9 ± 8.5	0 – 40	
Age at onset of epilepsy			
all (n = 170)	14.7 ± 3.7	5.8 – 26	
females	14.3 ± 4	5.8 – 26	
males	15.3 ± 3	9 – 24	
Age at onset of MJ (data reliable in 131/170)			
all (n = 131)	15.2 ± 3.8	7 – 35	
females	14.4 ± 3.5	7 – 26	
males	16.3 ± 4.1	9 – 35	
Age at onset of GTCS (data reliable in 140/151)			
all (n = 140)	16.4 ± 4.5	5.8 – 32	
females	16.3 ± 4.8	5.8 – 31	
males	16.6 ± 4.1	9 – 32	
Age at onset of TA (data reliable in 34/56)			
all (n = 34)	13.9 ± 3.4	7.5 – 22	
females	13.6 ± 4	8 – 22	
males	14.4 ± 2.5	7.5 – 18	
Seizure types	all	females	males
	n = 170	n = 104	n = 66
only MJ	15 (8.8%)	11 (10.6%)	4 (6.1%)
MJ + GTCS	99 (58.2%)	62 (59.6%)	37 (56.1%)
MJ + TA	4 (2.4%)	3 (2.9%)	1
MJ + GTCS + TA	52 (30.6%)	28 (26.9%)	24 (36.4%)
Photosensitivity	65 (38%)	48 (46%)	17 (26%)

This definition remains very unsatisfactory. Contrary to what is stated here, there is no clear continuum among the various conditions that are listed as IGEs (Genton, 1999); however, the main failing of this definition is the lack of any firm biological basis. Although it remains difficult to clearly define the limits of the concept of IGE, JME clearly belongs to that category of epilepsies, and is probably the most frequent type of IGE that is encountered in general neurological practice.

Three seizure types can be found in JME: myoclonic jerks (MJ), generalized tonic-clonic seizures (GTCS) and typical absences (TA). While MJ may remain the only seizure type in some patients (and in other subjects who probably never seek medical advice), they are very often associated with GTCS, less commonly with TA. There are no other seizure types in JME, except when, in selected instances, the usual seizures occur in clusters or in status, or when GTCS have an apparently lateralized onset. Although not entirely specific, this combination of seizures in an otherwise healthy person, the presence of identifiable triggering factors and fairly typical EEG changes makes the diagnosis of JME comparatively easy. The best approach to that diagnosis is syndromic: if taken together, all the elements from the patient's and his family's history, from the circumstances and clinical characteristics of seizures, from the EEG and from the evolution of the condition over the years (including the effect of the various medications that have been tried) bring about a firm diagnosis of JME.

JME: THE BACKGROUND

Prevalence

JME is a common type of epilepsy. It accounts for 2.8–11.9% of all epilepsies (review in Wolf, 1992a; Genton *et al.*, 1994). The prevalence in any given setting is clearly dependent on the type of recruitment, and the true prevalence among unselected epilepsies remains unclear, since many cases are un- or misdiagnosed. In the experience of a tertiary referral centre like the Centre Saint Paul in Marseille, comparatively benign and easily treatable forms of epilepsy tend to be underrepresented. Among 2811 consecutively referred patients seen between 1986 and 1997, the group of IGE represented 15.3% of all cases, and JME 26.7% of all IGE (4.1% of all epilepsies), preceding childhood absence epilepsy (23.3%); juvenile absence epilepsy (11%), photogenic epilepsy (9.1%) and awakening grand mal (6.2%). In our experience, which covers epilepsy patients of all age classes, JME is the most frequent form of IGE; in a less selective setting, it may well be the most frequent type of easily identifiable epileptic syndrome.

Family history and genetics

The genetic aspects of JME are complex, and are dealt with elsewhere in this volume. From a clinical point of view, however, it must be stressed that a family history of epilepsy should be weighed in as a diagnostic feature of JME, but that a majority of patients will appear as apparently isolated cases. In large family studies, undiagnosed cases may be detected by systematic interviews and/or systematic EEG recordings. In our patients, a family history of epilepsy in first and/or second-degree relatives was present in 72 cases/168 (43%; 2/170 cases were adopted in childhood and no family history is available). Epilepsy was present in more than one relative in 18 cases (10.7%). However, JME in other family members was ascertained in only 16 cases (9.5%).

Personal history

Like other forms of IGE, JME usually occurs in patients who have no significant prior history. In our series, a firm history of perinatal suffering was present in one case, and six patients were born prematurely without further complications; the patient with neonatal anoxia had mental retardation, diffuse brain atrophy on the computed tomography, and developed a typical form of JME after his delayed puberty, at age 18. Febrile seizures occurred in early childhood in 17/169 patients (10.1%); Janz (1991) reported a prevalence of 4.4%. Mental retardation was present in 11 cases (6.5%), of which two were considered severely, and nine mildly retarded. Psychiatric problems encountered in patients with JME will be discussed below. Two patients developed significant neurological problems after the onset of JME: one had multiple sclerosis, and one had a severe head trauma. A personal history, including potential factors of cerebral damage, is not considered significant for the diagnosis of JME (Wolf, 1992a).

Sex distribution and age-dependency (Figure 1)

We found a striking female predominance (61%, sex ratio = 1.56) among our patients. This has already been noted in recent studies, but others reported a male predominance (33 vs 20 females, Delgado-Escueta and Enrile-Bacsal, 1984). However, those who used to stress the equal sex distribution (Janz, 1969; Tsuboi, 1977) now admit a slight female predominance (Janz and Durner, 1998). The sex of the patients has little influence on the clinical course and symptomatology of JME. Seizures, and especially MJ, tend to occur at an earlier age in female patients (median: 14 vs 16 years), but this may simply reflect the faster development of pubertal maturation in girls.

The onset of seizures in JME is clearly an age-related phenomenon (Figure 1). There is a striking peak around the age of puberty, i.e. 12–14 years in girls, vs 14–16 in boys. The onset of JME is practically limited to the second decade of life, with a clearly unimodal distribution, with 11 cases (6.5%) beginning before the age of 10, and 17 cases (10%) at age 20 or more. None of the patients with early onset had a typical form of childhood absence epilepsy and evolved into JME secondarily. Onset in elderly patients remains anecdotal (Gram et al., 1988). There is apparently no influence of the age of onset on severity and long-term evolution. Among 22 patients with onset at age 10 or below, we only noted that 50% had a photoparoxysmal response on their EEG (vs 38% of the whole sample), and 50% had TAs (vs 38% of the whole

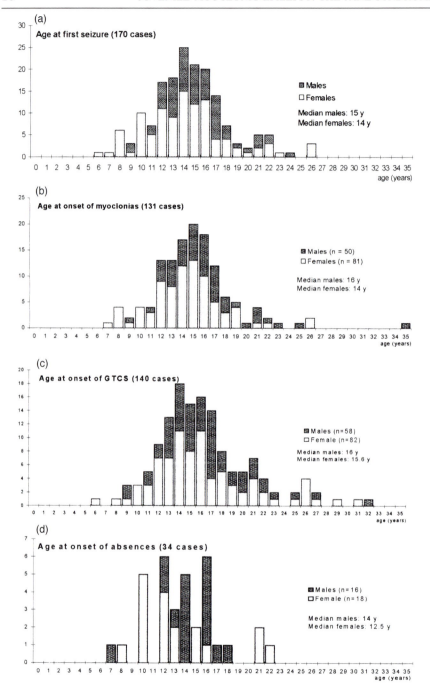

Figure 1. Age at onset according to sex: (a) first seizure; (b) onset of myoclonias; (c) onset of generalized tonic-clonic seizures (GTCS); (d) onset of absences. Age at onset was slightly lower in females, especially for myoclonic jerks and absences.

sample). Patients with onset at age 20 or later cannot be distinguished from the whole sample in terms of seizure type or association of seizure types.

Circumstances at referral and triggering factors

In most cases, patients will come to their physician after the first GTCS, and have a previous history of isolated MJ. The first GTCS has usually been triggered by a specific circumstance, or an accumulation of circumstances, including sleep deprivation, excessive intake of alcohol, stress, fatigue, and, in some girls or young women, the menstrual period. According to Pedersen and Petersen (1998), the most common precipitating factors are sleep deprivation (84%), stress (70%), and alcohol consumption (51%). Typical examples of circumstances leading to the first GTCS can be quoted: in a 14 year-old girl, night-time bus journey from skiing holidays, with arrival at her home town and abrupt awakening at 3 a.m.; in a 19 year-old man, early awakening one morning after three nights of 'fiesta' following a successful examination; in a 20 year-old woman, referral on 1 January, after she had spent the evening drinking champagne with her family, and the night dancing and drinking in a discotheque with her boyfriend. In a specific setting, other precipitating factors may be involved, like illicit drugs, drug withdrawal or psychotropic medications such as amitriptyline (Resor and Resor, 1990). The role played by alcohol consumption has been stressed by several authors: it was implicated in 40% of their patients by Janz and Christian (1957), and in 30% by Penry et al. (1989).

However, the precise diagnosis of JME is rarely made at that point, unless the patient is quickly referred to a specialized epilepsy clinic. They usually are, but very late, and may be referred at that late stage for a variety of reasons. Among the 170 patients we recently evaluated, the diagnoses made by the referring physician could be ascertained in 137 cases, as shown in Table 2.

Diagnostic delay and misdiagnosis

It is thus clear that JME remains underdiagnosed. In our recent series, the mean delay between onset of seizures and diagnosis of JME was nearly 8

Table 2. Diagnoses made by referring physicians (137 cases).

JME and/or IGE	22	(16%)
Petit mal epilepsy	2	(1.5%)
Epilepsy, no precise diagnosis	70	(51%)
Focal epilepsy	10	(7.3%)
Post-traumatic epilepsy	1	(0.7%)
Panic attacks	4	(3%)
Other non-epileptic events	28	(20.5%)

years (Table 1). Several factors may lead to such delay. Clinical factors include unreported jerks, reported asymmetrical or unilateral jerks, reported versive onset of a GTCS, and (most importantly) lack of knowledge of the syndrome by clinicians (Panayiotopoulos *et al.*, 1991; Lancman *et al.*, 1994). The EEG may also be misleading, either because it fails to show abnormalities (leading to the diagnosis of non-epileptic events, or of an undetermined form of epilepsy), or because it shows asymmetrical or even focal changes (leading to a diagnosis of focal epilepsy) (Aliberti *et al.*, 1994; Genton *et al.*, 1995; Lombroso, 1997; So *et al.*, 1998). Misdiagnosis may have dramatic consequences, as some patients will be aggravated by inadequate drugs for many years (Kivity and Rechtman, 1995; Atakli *et al.*, 1998).

JME: THE CLINICAL SYNDROME

Myoclonic jerks

The major diagnostic feature is represented by MJ, occurring preferentially within 5–30 min after awakening, especially when the night has been short or the awakening sudden. They typically lead to incidents during breakfast (the spoon, or the cup is thrown away), or during ablutions (the patient cuts himself with the razor). They can also happen upon awakening from an afternoon nap. They may also occur in an isolated manner, during daytime, and, especially in some patients, in the evening period of relaxation. The MJ are of varying intensity: at the maximum, they may cause the patient to fall; at the minimum, they are nearly subclinical, or subjective, reported as 'an internal electric shock'. They are often referred to as clumsiness, or tremor; they are also often reported as unilateral, implying only the leading hand, for instance. They are usually not accompanied by loss of consciousness, although some patients feel and describe a sort of numbness, especially when the MJ occur in brief clusters. Patients may become accustomed to such MJ, and consider them as minor troubles, unworthy of chronic treatment, even after an accurate diagnosis has been proposed when medical advice has been sought.

These MJ remain the only seizure type in few patients (15/170, 8.8% in our experience), and are the first seizures in most cases. They tend to occur sporadically, sometimes repeatedly over several minutes, in short irregular series, and not every day. Triggering factors play a major role in their appearance. Patients with isolated jerks may represent a minor form of JME (Jain *et al.*, 1997). Myoclonic status, or prolonged episodes of jerks, may occur in some patients (7.3% in the series of Salas-Puig *et al.*, 1990; only three cases, or 2%, in the present series): the most serious episodes of myoclonic status may be related to inadequate treatment of JME, or to abrupt withdrawal of antiepileptic drugs (AEDs).

Generalized tonic-clonic seizures

GTCS are found in a large majority of cases (88.8% in our series), and are often the symptom that leads to the first medical intervention, even though they may occur several years after the first MJ. Our data are in accordance with those of former series (Janz, 1969; Tsuboi, 1977; Obeid and Panayiotopoulos, 1988) (80–95%). GTCS are often preceded by a series of massive myoclonic jerks – thus being in fact clonic-tonic-clonic seizures (Delgado-Escueta and Enrile-Bacsal, 1984), and share the same circadian distribution and triggering factors as the jerks. In JME, GTCS are usually reported as very long, dramatic and tend to leave a long-lasting fatigue. They are not very frequent (one per year or less), unless particular elements of the patient's lifestyle play an aggravating role, or when inadequate drugs are given. They may however be frequent, and debilitating, in selected patients who do follow medical advice and treatment, or during a particular period, usually during adolescence or early adulthood. The unusual occurrence of versive, or even circling seizures, presumably at the onset of GTCS, has been reported recently in various forms of IGE, including patients with JME (Topcuoglu *et al.*, 1997; Aguglia *et al.*, 1999).

Absences

Absences were not considered a major feature in the original description of JME; they occur in a minority of patients (56/170 cases, 33% in our series), but may be underestimated as they may escape the attention of the patient's entourage and remain ignored by the patient himself. Their existence in JME is however increasingly recognized: they were found in 10% of the patients by Janz (1969); 14% by Tsuboi (1977), 18% by Obeid and Panayiotopoulos (1988). In JME, TA are infrequent, occurring typically less than several times per week, and are usually short. They are apparently associated with an earlier onset of JME (Table 1). A more systematic approach and a closer description of the features of absences in JME was made by Panayiotopoulos *et al.* in 1989, who showed that TA may be found in as many as 38% of JME patients when systematic, long-term video-EEG monitoring is used. Absence status may occur in adults with JME, but remains a fairly uncommon situation (Agathonikou *et al.*, 1998).

Photosensitivity

Some patients may experience MJ, or even GTCS triggered by visual stimuli (television and videogames, but also stroboscopic lights in discos, or intense sunlight), in association with the spontaneously occurring attacks. However, clinical photosensitivity remains quite uncommon in JME (5% in our earlier work (Genton *et al.*, 1994)), and probably has been neglected to some extent. However, the presence of a photoparoxysmal response provoked by intermittent light stimulation during the EEG recording is much more frequent: we found such responses in 38% of the JME patients, and, in accordance with the higher prevalence of photosensitivity among females, with a much lower prevalence among males (26% vs 48%).

Combinations of seizures

Most patients will experience a combination of seizures, with relatively frequent jerks and infrequent GTCS being the most common combination (58.2% in our series). There does not appear to be a specific, sex-linked association of seizures, although male patients are more likely to have all three seizure types in combination than females (36.4 vs 26.9%). As already stated, a sizeable proportion of JME cases (including relatives of patients of JME probands) may experience only infrequent jerks and may totally escape medical attention and diagnosis. A small minority of patients (2.4%) will experience the uncommon combination of MJ and TA. Thus JME is a mixed seizure disorder, but, unlike other epileptic syndromes that qualify as such (e.g. the Lennox–Gastaut syndrome), it is not a severe condition.

Circadian distribution of seizures: chronosensitivity

The circadian distribution of the seizures is one of the major clinical characteristics of JME. This was already clear to Janz and Christian in 1957. Touchon *et al.* (1982) stressed, in their systematic survey, the existence of a peak of occurrence of seizures at awakening, in the morning in most cases, during intermediate nocturnal awakenings, or after an afternoon nap in others, with a lesser peak during the evening relaxation period. The polyspike-waves recorded on the EEG follow a similar pattern, with a cluster of discharges after awakening, and a relative build-up of discharges during the nocturnal sleep period (Figure 2).

Psychiatric problems in JME patients

JME is a stable condition and is not associated with mental or neurological deterioration. According to Janz and Christian (1957), JME patients often have an unstable personality, which may lead to social maladjustment, inadequate lifestyle and low compliance; such findings rely on clinical experience, but are difficult to quantify. It has been suggested that some of such behavioural problems might be linked to frontal lobe dysfunction (Devinsky *et al.*, 1997). Like other forms of idiopathic epilepsies, JME may be fortuitously associated with mental retardation and/or psychiatric problems. In our series,

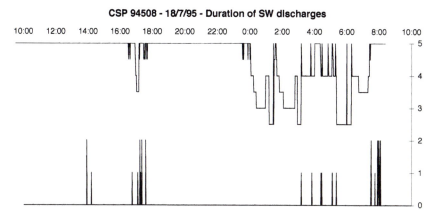

Figure 2. Circadian distribution of spike-waves (SW) in a 38 year-old untreated male patient with JME since age 15: (top) sleep stages; (bottom) duration of SW (scale from 1 to 5 seconds, on the right). Note the striking increase after awakening, both from the afternoon nap and from the night's sleep. Also note the scarcity of discharges during the daytime and during the first portion of the night. This patient had been on valproate for many years, and decided to stop medication at age 36. Two years later, he came back for re-evalution, and complained of frequent jerks in the morning. No GTCS had recurred, but the patient resumed his medication.

we found the following psychiatric problems: severe mental retardation (1), pervasive developmental disorder (2), tic disorder (1), enuresis (1), psychosis (5), depressive disorder (3), generalized anxiety (3), anorexia nervosa (2); personality disorder (24), including borderline personality in 11 cases. It must be noted that very different psychiatric diagnoses were made, and most of these disorders have no apparent logical link with JME. However, the high number of patients with personality disorders (24, i.e. 14% of our sample) is striking. Although such 'difficult' patients may be overrepresented in this series, these findings clearly indicate that further research is necessary.

Associated medical disorders

There are no medical disorders that are significantly associated with JME. In our series, one patient manifested an aggravation of seizures and was diagnosed as having hypothyroidism: thyroid replacement therapy quickly led to improvement of seizure control. We also know middle-aged patients with JME (not included in this series) with diabetes mellitus, and some GTCS may have been precipitated by hypoglycaemia. Hyperthyroidism has also been reported as an aggravating factor in JME (Su *et al.*, 1993).

More puzzling are recent reports on JME associated with focal epilepsy (Diehl *et al.*, 1998; Koutroumanidis *et al.*, 1999). Two patients are described, who were surgically treated for intractable temporal lobe epilepsy, apparently with success, but had persisting clinical and EEG symptoms of JME after the procedure.

Neuroimaging

Modern neuroimaging techniques (CT, magnetic resonance imaging (MRI)) are not necessary in patients with JME. Serratosa and Delgado-Escueta (1993) report that MRI and PET studies were consistently normal in their patients. In our series, 82 patients were investigated, mostly prior to referral to our centres: 22 had MRI, 75 had CT scans, and 15 had both. Four patients had abnormal MRI and significant neurological problems unrelated to JME: multiple sclerosis (1), traumatic brain lesion after severe head trauma (2), birth trauma with diffuse brain atrophy (1). Among the other 78 patients, nine had abnormal findings: arachnoid cyst (3), mild ventricular enlargement (3), mild diffuse cortical atrophy (1), septum lucidum cyst (1), mild MRI hyper-signal in the left temporal lobe (1). Such findings can be considered coincidental. More importantly, these findings confirm that the diagnosis of JME may stand, even in the presence of morphological abnormalities in the brain.

Evolution and prognosis

JME was described as 'benign juvenile myoclonic epilepsy' (Wolf, 1985) before the present denomination was universally adopted; the fact that 'benign' was dropped points to a mitigated appraisal of the severity of this condition. The main factor that made experts reconsider the 'benignity' of JME was the fact that, contrary to the clearly benign childhood onset idiopathic focal epilepsies, that have an age-dependent expression and constantly remit before puberty, JME tends to be a life-long condition. Even after years of full seizure control, the discontinuation of drug therapy leads to a very high rate of relapse, probably close to 90% (Janz et al., 1983; Delgado-Escueta and Enrile-Bacsal, 1984; Baruzzi et al., 1988; Canevini et al., 1992). In such well-controlled patients, however, treatment with low-dose valproate (VPA) becomes an option (De Toffol and Autret, 1996). However, the evolution of JME in middle-aged and elderly patients has not been studied fully. Our clinical experience shows that patients above the age of 40 tend to have a milder clinical expression of their condition, but very few patients have been followed over many years and precise data are lacking.

Another factor is the realization that some patients may have, transiently or permanently, a severe form of JME. Although the symptoms are usually abated during pregnancy (Asconapé and Penry, 1984), there is often an increased risk of seizures after delivery, due to the usual lack of sleep associated with the first weeks of breast feeding. Seizures may be increased in periods of stress, or may represent a significant handicap for vocational orientation. Some forms of JME may be truly drug-resistant. In our series, we found that among 155 patients who had been followed for at least one year, 39 (25%) had persisting seizures. Among these, 15 were considered to be pseudo-resistant, due to grossly inadequate lifestyle (4), lack of compliance (8) or treatment with inadequate AEDs (3). However, 24 patients (15.5%) had persisting seizures in spite of an adequate lifestyle and of adequate medication. The factors associated with drug resistance were: presence of mental retardation (21% of resistant vs 3% of non-resistant cases), presence of psychiatric problems (58.3% vs 19%), presence of the association of all three seizure types (62.5% vs 28.4%). Three patients died during follow-up: one died during sleep (history: suicide attempts, anorexia nervosa); one was found dead in her home, presumably after a GTCS (history: moderate mental retardation, alcoholism, neuroleptic treatment); one died while in the toilet, presumably during a seizure (history: severe mental retardation, psychosis, neuroleptic treatment). Thus a few JME patients with several risk factors, among which are mental retardation and psychiatric disorders, are at risk of sudden death.

Thus JME, which remains a benign condition in most patients, may be severe in a minority of cases. Most studies have stressed that 80–90% of the patients are fully controlled under adequate treatment, but this leaves more than 10% with persisting, often debilitating seizures.

The effect of antiepileptic medication

JME is characterized by a specific pharmacological sensitivity: JME is controlled by certain AEDs, but may be aggravated by others. In 1957, Janz and Christian had already shown that a 'predominantly barbituric' regimen controlled 86% of the patients, while a regimen containing predominantly phenytoin (PHT) controlled only 67% and left 33% unchanged or worsened. Phenobarbital and primidone were thus the treatment of choice, until VPA monotherapy was shown to control as many as 86% of JME patients (Penry et al., 1989); in our series, 84.5% of the patients followed for at least one year were likewise totally controlled. Other drugs that have been shown to help control JME are clonazepam, which may be used in cotherapy with VPA (Obeid and Panayiotopoulos, 1989), acetazolamide (Resor and Resor, 1990) and methsuximide (Hurst, 1996). Among the newer AEDs, those that appear to be useful are lamotrigine (Buchanan, 1996; Wallace, 1998), often used in combination with VPA, and topiramate (Kellett et al., 1999).

However, much emphasis has been put recently on the aggravating effect of AEDs, and JME is a clear candidate for such paradoxical effects of medical prescriptions (Bauer, 1996; Perucca et al., 1998; Genton and McMenamin, 1998). In our series, PHT was not very efficient: among 18 patients exposed to PHT, eight did not notice a change in seizure frequency, six were aggravated and only four were improved. PHT may be pushed to high doses in refractory JME patients, and may thus clearly exacerbate MJ (Kivity and Rechtman, 1995); PHT exacerbated MJ in two of three of the JME patients reported by Sözüer *et al.* (1996). However, carbamazepine (CBZ) seems to be the drug with the most pronounced aggravating effect: in our series, it aggravated nearly 68% of the patients exposed to it (19/28). This paradoxical effect was reported by others, in similar proportions, and some patients experienced myoclonic status on CBZ (Kivity and Rechtman, 1995). Some authors still advocate the use of CBZ in selected cases. Oxcarbazepine, which is closely related to CBZ, may have a similar aggravating effect. Among newer AEDs, VGB had been prescribed in only one case in our series, and apparently triggered, when added to CBZ, a mixed status epilepticus of myoclonias and absences; however, Pedersen *et al.* (1985) noted that VGB produced a 50% reduction of seizures in three JME patients. There are no data on the efficiency of gabapentin or tiagabine in JME, but it is suspected that these AEDs might also provoke aggravation.

It thus appears that JME has a characteristic pharmacological sensitivity, which it may share with other IGEs. This sensitivity contributes to its clinical definition, and sets it clearly apart, for instance, from frontal lobe epilepsies. Given the high rate of misdiagnosis in patients with JME, an inadequate choice of drug may, by leading to exacerbation of MJ and GTCS (and of the typical EEG changes), facilitate the diagnosis of JME.

THE LIMITS OF JME

As stated repeatedly above, the main problem with JME remains the fact that it is often un- or misdiagnosed. There are few circumstances in which JME is overdiagnosed, and the most difficult questions that remain open to discussion concern the boundaries between JME and other types of IGE. The complexity of this situation is illustrated in Figure 3. However, it should be stressed here that this discussion may be important for basic scientists and geneticists, but has comparatively little influence on the clinical management of JME patients.

JME may be diagnosed incorrectly at the initial stages of progressive myoclonus epilepsies of the Unverricht–Lundborg type or of the Lafora type (Roger *et al.*, 1992): however, the specific clinical and EEG traits of these conditions will quickly lead to a correction of the diagnosis. A newly reported syndrome of benign, adult-age onset syndrome of progressive myoclonus with some GTCS has been reported recently from Japan (Okino, 1997). However, MJ appear to be permanent in this condition, there is a strong genetic background suggesting mendelian transmission, and the EEG characteristics

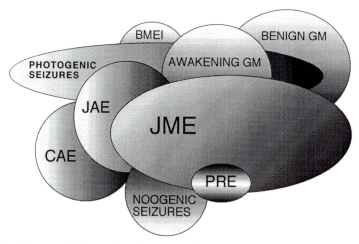

Figure 3. A constellation of epileptic syndromes around JME. (BMEI, benign myoclonic epilepsy in infancy; CAE, childhood absence epilepsy; GM, grand mal; JAE, juvenile absence epilepsy; PRE, primary reading epilepsy).

of JME are not present. Some focal epilepsies of frontal lobe origin may be mistaken for JME, or *vice versa*, but the evolution is generally much more severe, and the recording of seizures on the EEG will easily correct the diagnosis (Roger and Bureau, 1992). A clinical picture that strongly resembles JME has been reported as 'senile myoclonic epilepsy' in elderly Down syndrome patients who become demented (Genton and Paglia, 1994), and may also occur in Alzheimer patients, but such cases are rarely well-documented, and the setting is clearly different from that of JME.

Our present knowledge leads us to assume that there is no biological continuum between the different syndromes of IGE (Roger *et al.*, 1994). However, JME is at the crossroads of several syndromes that are included among IGEs. Such syndromes are separated according to the main seizure type involved, i.e. TA, MJ or GTCS.

Childhood absence epilepsy (CAE), in its typical pyknoleptic form can easily be separated from JME, on clinical, neurophysiological and genetic grounds, in spite of reports of cases evolving from CAE to JME (Rabe, 1961). Janz reported in 1969 that 4.6% of all CAE patients evolved into JME. Juvenile absence epilepsy (JAE), on the contrary, is more difficult to detach from JME: according to the classical descriptions (review in Wolf, 1992b), absences are not pyknoleptic, MJ can occur, GTCS are frequent, and the seizures tend to persist into adulthood. In some patients with JAE, TA may occur randomly, while JM and/or GTCS may be provoked by the same triggering factors as in JME. According to Wolf (1992b), JAE may be considered to be an 'intermediate syndrome' between CAE and JME; however, there is no clinical evidence that patients may go from CAE in childhood through JAE in late childhood and into JME at adolescence. Besides the two classical forms of absence epilepsies, there are other types that may, in some cases, overlap with JME: absences that are strictly provoked by intermittent light stimulation (e.g. by a TV screen) and that seem to occur on a strong genetic, autosomal dominant basis (Grinspan *et al.*, 1992), the syndrome of absences with eyelid myoclonias, that has also many of the characteristics of a photogenic epilepsy (Jeavons, 1977), and in general all forms of absence epilepsy with a strong photosensitivity.

Among the IGEs, there is a very early-onset form that is characterized, just as JME, by the occurrence of MJ and frequent photosensitivity: in this benign myoclonic epilepsy in infancy (BMEI, Dravet and Bureau, 1981), there are however no other seizure types involved, and the seizures often remit spontaneously during childhood. A later-onset type of BMEI has been described by Guerrini *et al.* (1994) but it also apparently remits in late childhood, before the usual onset of JME. In our series, we found no evident overlap between the classical or late variant type of BMEI and JME, since patients with early onset of JME, before age 10, tended to have TA and GTCS besides JM. But a very early onset of MJ in JME has been reported, and an overlap is clearly possible. MJ are also the predominant ictal manifestation in patients who experience seizures triggered by intellectual processes, described as 'noogenic epilepsies' by Gastaut in 1988, and as 'praxis-induced seizures' by Inoue *et al.* in 1994. Primary reading epilepsy, which used to be considered a specific entity related to the idiopathic focal epilepsies, is close to JME in many cases, although it is still considered a separate syndrome (Mayer and Wolf, 1999).

There is only one recognized syndrome of IGE that has GTCS as the main and most characteristic seizure type, i. e. 'awakening grand mal' (AGM) (Wolf, 1992c). In AGM, both TA and MJ may occur, the former quite often, the latter quite rarely; there is a slight male predominance, and the age at onset ranges from early childhood into adulthood. In fact, many cases of IGE with GTCS have been ascribed to the syndrome of AGM in spite of the absence of a clear relationship between the seizures and the offset of the sleep period (Roger *et al.*, 1994). Many of such cases, that present usually with very infrequent GTCS, without clear triggering factors, might be better described as 'benign grand mal', whether the onset is in adults (Oller-Daurella and Sorel, 1989), or in earlier age classes. Probands with JME often have among their first- and second-degree relatives such patients, and in such cases the 'grand mal' epilepsy might represent a minor form of JME.

CONCLUSIONS

Juvenile myoclonic epilepsy is both a frequent and a very characteristic epileptic syndrome, and JME is increasingly recognized, correctly diagnosed

Table 3. Diagnostic features of JME.

Genetic background
    idiopathic generalized epilepsies in the family
    apparently isolated cases are common

No significant personal history
    rare exceptions: may occur in patients with neurological deficits
                may follow earlier-onset epilepsy

Female predominance (moderate)

Associated seizure types
    myoclonic jerks (MJ) in all patients
    GTCS in most, often triggering medical intervention
    infrequent absences possible
    episodes of status possible, triggered by inadequate drugs

Onset around puberty
    from late childhood into early adulthood
    apparent onset (first GTCS) may be different from real onset (MJ)

Triggering factors of seizures
    sleep deprivation
    alcohol intake
    photic stimulation from the environment (more in females)
    other factors possible (stress, fatigue, premenstrual syndrome)

Chronodependency
    a major peak of clinical manifestations at awakening from sleep
    a lesser evening peak

Associated symptoms
    none in most patients
    mild to moderate psychopathology possible

EEG
    irregular, fast polyspike-waves (PSW) on the interictal EEG
    myoclonic jerks are always associated with PSW discharges

Pharmacological sensitivity
    responds to a limited number of drugs
        valproate is the drug of choice
    symptoms may be aggravated by several drugs
        (carbamazepine most frequently responsible)

Pharmacodependency
    relapse after cessation of therapy in most cases
    appears to be a life-long condition

Overall prognosis
    remains a benign condition in most patients
    may be problematic in some cases (e.g. with associated psychiatric problems)

and treated with the adequate regimen. The main distinctive clinical traits of JME are summarized in Table 2. The typical, full-blown clinical and electrophysiological picture of JME probably represents a 'hard core' at the fringe of which some phenotypic variants, or transitional forms occur. The closest relationships are with the various syndromes of IGE, and with photogenic epilepsies. In its most typical forms, JME might well be a disease, with only slight variations in age-dependency and prognosis. However, given the absence of a firm biological or genetic basis, and the existence of bordering epileptic entities that share many, but not all of its features, it should still be regarded as a syndrome. It will probably take some time before the Janz syndrome becomes a disease!

In clinical practice, JME can be easily and firmly diagnosed by careful interview with the patient and the witnesses of the attacks, and by the EEG, with the help, if necessary, of long-term EEG-video monitoring using sleep and/or sleep deprivation recordings. Here is a form of epilepsy that can be treated to the patient's satisfaction in most cases, even if we still do not have an intimate understanding of its aetiology. When taking a patient with JME into our care, we can already act rationally with today's diagnostic and therapeutic tools, and also help the basic scientists and geneticists in their quest for the ultimate explanation of JME.

ACKNOWLEDGEMENT

Dr Philippe Gélisse's research was supported by a research grant from the French League Against Epilepsy and the Janssen-Cilag company.

REFERENCES:

Agathonikou, A., Panayiotopoulos, C.P., Giannakodimos, S. Koutroumanidis, M. (1998). Typical absence status in adults: diagnostic and syndromic considerations. *Epilepsia* **39**, 1265–1276.

Aguglia, U., Gambardella, A., Le Piane, E., Messina, D., Russo, C., Oliveri, R.L., Zappia, M. and Quattrone, A. (1999). Idiopathic generalized epilepsies with versive or circling seizures. *Acta Neurol Scand* **99**, 219–224.

Aliberti, V., Grünewald, R.A. and Panayiotopoulos, C.P. (1994). Focal EEG abnormalities in juvenile myoclonic epilepsy. *Epilepsia* **35**, 297–301.

Asconapé, J. and Penry, J.K. (1984). Some clinical and EEG aspects of benign juvenile myoclonic epilepsy. *Epilepsia* **25**, 108–114.

Atakli, D., Sözüer, D., Atay, T., Baybas S. and Arpaci, B. (1998). Misdiagnosis and treatment in juvenile myoclonic epilepsy. *Seizure* **7**, 63–66.

Baruzzi, A., Procaccianti, G., Tinuper, P. and Lugaresi, E. (1988). Antiepileptic drug withdrawal in childhood epilepsies: preliminary results of a prospective study. In: Faienza, C. and Prati, G.L. (Eds), *Diagnostic and Therapeutic Problems in Pediatric Epileptology*. Elsevier, Amsterdam, pp. 117–123.

Bauer, J. (1996). Seizure-inducing effect of antiepileptic drugs: a review. *Acta Neurol Scand* **94**, 367–377.

Buchanan, N. (1996). The use of lamotrigine in juvenile myoclonic epilepsy. *Seizure* **5**, 149–151.

Canevini, M.P., Mai, R., Di-Marco, C. *et al.* (1992) Juvenile myoclonic epilepsy of Janz: clinical observations in 60 patients. *Seizure* **1**, 291–298.

Commission on Classification and Terminology of the International League Against Epilepsy (1989). Proposal for revised classification of epilepsies and epileptic syndromes. *Epilepsia* **30**, 389–399.

Delgado-Escueta, A.V. and Enrile-Bacsal, F. (1984). Juvenile myoclonic epilepsy of Janz. *Neurology* **34**, 285–24.

De Toffol, B. and Autret, A. (1996). Treatment of juvenile myoclonic epilepsy with low-dose sodium valproate. *Rev Neurol* **152**, 708–710.

Devinsky, O., Gershengorn, J., Brown, E., Perrine, K., Vazquez, B. and Luciano, D. (1997). Frontal functions in juvenile myoclonic epilepsy. *Neuropsychiatry Neuropsychol Behav Neurol* **10**, 243–246.

Diehl, B., Wyllie, E., Rothner, A.D. and Bingamen, W. (1998). Worsening seizures after surgery for focal epilepsy due to emergence of primary generalized epilepsy. *Neurology* **51**, 1178–1180.

Dinner, D.S., Lüders, H., Morris, H.H. and Lesser, R.P. (1987). Juvenile myoclonic epilepsy. In: Lüders, H. and Lesser, R.P. (Eds), *Epilepsy: Electroclinical Syndromes*. Springer Verlag, Berlin, pp. 131–149.

Dravet, C. and Bureau, M. (1981). L'épilepsie myoclonique bénigne du nourrisson. *Rev EEG Neurophysiol* **11**, 438–444.

Gastaut, H. (1988). Synopsis and conclusion of the international colloquium on reflex seizures and epilepsies. In: Beaumanoir, A., Gastaut, H. and Naquet, R. (Eds), *Reflex Seizures and Reflex Epilepsies*. Editions Médecine et Hygiène, Geneva, pp. 497–507.

Genton, P. (1999). Limites du concept d'épilepsie généralisé et idiopathique. *Rev Neurol* **155**, 121–128.

Genton, P. and McMenamin, J. (1998). Can antiepileptic drugs aggravate epilepsy? *Epilepsia* (suppl 3), 29 pp.

Genton, P. and Paglia, G. (1994). Épilepsie myoclonique sénile? Myoclonies épileptiques d'apparition tardive dans le syndrome de Down. *Epilepsies* **6**, 5–11.

Genton, P., Salas Puig, J., Tunon, A., Lahoz, C. and Gonzalez Sanchez, M. (1994). Juvenile myoclonic epilepsy and related syndromes: clinical and neurophysiological aspects. In: Malafosse, A., Genton, P., Hirsch, E., Marescaux, C., Broglin, D. and Bernasconi, R. (Eds), *Idiopathic Generalized Epilepsies: Clinical, Experimental and Genetic Aspects*. John Libbey, London, pp. 253–265.

Genton, P., Gonzales Sanchez, M.D.S., Saltarelli, A., Bureau, M., Dravet, C. and Roger, J. (1995). Aspects trompeurs de l'EEG standard dans l'épilepsie myoclonique juvénile: étude rétrospective de 56 cas consécutifs. *Neurophysiol Clin* **25**, 285–290.

Gram, L., Alving, J., Sagild, J.C. and Dam, M. (1988). Juvenile myoclonic epilepsy in unexpected age groups. *Epilepsy Res* **2**, 137–140.

Grinspan, A., Hirsch, E., Malafosse, A. and Marescaux, C. (1992). Épilepsie-absences photosensible familiale: un nouveau syndrome? *Epilepsies* **4**, 245–250.

Grünewald, R.A. and Panayiotopoulos, D.P. (1993). Juvenile myoclonic epilepsy: a review. *Arch Neurol* **50**, 594–598.

Guerrini, R., Dravet, C., Gobbi, G., Ricci, S. and Dulac, O. (1994). Idiopathic generalized epilepsies with myoclonus in infancy and childhood. In: Malafosse, A., Genton, P., Hirsch, E., Marescaux, C., Broglin, D. and Bernasconi, R. (Eds), *Idiopathic Generalized Epilepsies: Clinical, Experimental and Genetic Aspects*. John Libbey, London, pp. 267–280.

Hurst, D.L. (1996). Methsuximide therapy of juvenile myoclonic epilepsy. *Seizure* **5**, 47–50.

Inoue, Y., Seino, M., Kubota, H., Yamakaku, K., Tanaka, M. and Yagi, K. (1994). Epilepsy with praxis-induced seizures. In: Wolf, P. (Ed.), *Epileptic Seizures and Syndromes*. John Libbey, London, pp. 81–92.

Jain, S., Padma, M.V. and Maheshwari, M.C. (1997). Occurrence of only myoclonic jerks in juvenile myoclonic epilepsy. *Acta Neurol Scand* **95**, 263–267.

Janz, D. (1969). *Die Epilepsien*. Thieme Verlag, Stuttgart.

Janz, D. (1991). Juvenile myoclonic epilepsy. In: Dam, M. and Gram, L. (Eds), *Comprehensive Epileptology*. Raven Press, New York, pp. 171–185.

Janz, D. and Christian, W. (1957). Impulsiv petit-mal. *Dtsch Z. Nervenheilk* **176**, 346–386.

Janz, D. and Durner, M. (1998). Juvenile myoclonic epilepsy. In: Engel, J. and Pedley, T.A. (Eds), *Epilepsy: A Comprehensive Textbook*. Lippincott-Raven, Philadelphia, pp. 2389–2400.

Janz, D., Kern, A., Mössinger, H.-J. and Puhlmann, U. (1983). Rücksall-Prognon nach Reduktion bei Epilepsibehandlung. *Nervenarzt* **54**, 525–529.

Jeavons, P.M. (1977). Nosological problems of myoclonic epilepsies in childhood and adolescence. *Dev Med Child Neurol* **19**, 3–8.

Kellett, M.V., Smith, D.F., Stockton, P.A. and Chadwick, D.W. (1999). Topiramate in clinical practice: first year's post-licensing experience in a specialist epilepsy clinic. *J Neurol Neurosurg Psychiatry* **66**, 759–763.

Kivity, S. and Rechtman, E. (1995). Juvenile myoclonic epilepsy: serious consequences due to pitfalls in diagnosis and management. *Epilepsia* **36**, S66.

Koutroumanidis, M., Hennessy, M.J., Elwes, R.D., Binnie, C.D. and Polkey, C.E. (1999). Coexistence of temporal lobe and idiopathic generalized epilepsies. *Neurology* **53**, 490–495.

Lancman, M.E., Asconapé, J.J. and Penry, J.K. (1994). Clinical and EEG asymmetries in juvenile myoclonic epilepsy. *Epilepsia* **35**, 302–306.

Lombroso, C.T. (1997). Consistent EEG focalities detected in subjects with primary generalized epilepsies monitored for two decades. *Epilepsia* **38**, 797–812.

Mayer, T. and Wolf, P. (1999). Reading epilepsy: clinical and genetic background. In: Berkovic, S., Genton, P., Hirsch, E. and Picard, F. (Eds), *Genetics of Focal Epilepsies*. John Libbey, London, pp. 159–168.

Obeid, T. and Panayiotopoulos, C.P. (1988). Juvenile myoclonic epilepsy: a study in Saudi Arabia. *Epilepsia* **29**, 280–282.

Obeid, T. and Panayiotopoulos, C.P. (1989). Clonazepam in juvenile myoclonic epilepsy. *Epilepsia* **30**, 603–606.

Okino, S. (1997). Familial benign myoclonus epilepsy of adult onset: a previously unrecognized myoclonic disorder. *J Neurol Sci* **145**, 113–118.

Oller-Daurella, L. and Sorel, L. (1989). L'épilepsie grand mal bénigne de l'adulte. *Acta Neurol Belg* **89**, 38–45.

Panayiotopoulos, C.P., Obeid, T. and Waheed, G. (1989). Absences in juvenile myoclonic epilepsy: a clinical video-EEG study. *Ann Neurol* **25**, 391–397.

Panayiotopoulos, C.P., Tahan, R. and Obeid, T. (1991). Juvenile myoclonic epilepsy: factors of errors involved in the diagnosis and treatment. *Epilepsia* **32**, 672–676.

Pedersen, S.B. and Petersen, K.A. (1998). Juvenile myoclonic epilepsy: clinical and EEG features. *Acta Neurol Scand* **97**, 160–163.

Pedersen, S.A., Klosterskov, P., Gram, L. and Dam, M. (1985). Long-term study of gamma-vinyl GABA in the treatment of epilepsy. *Acta Neurol Scand* **72**, 295–298.

Penry, J.K., Dean, J.C. and Riela, A.R. (1989). Juvenile myoclonic epilepsy: long-term response to therapy. *Epilepsia* **30** (suppl 4), 19–23.

Perucca, E., Gram, L., Avanzini, G. and Dulac, O. (1998). Antiepileptic drugs as a cause of worsening seizures. *Epilepsia* **39**, 5–17.

Rabe, F. (1961) Zum Wechsel des Anfallscharakters epileptischer Anfälle. *Dtsch Z. Nervenheilk* **182**, 201–230.

Resor, S.R. and Resor, L.D. (1990). The neuropharmacology of juvenile myoclonic epilepsy. *Clin Neuropharmacol* **13**, 465–491.

Roger, J. and Bureau, M. (1992). Distinctive characteristics of frontal lobe epilepsy versus idiopathic generalized epilepsy. In: Chauvel, P., Delgado-Escueta, A.V., Halgren, E. and Bancaud, J. (Eds), *Frontal lobe seizures and epilepsies. Advances in Neurology, Vol. 57.* Raven Press, New York, pp. 399–410.

Roger, J., Genton, P., Bureau, M. and Dravet, C. (1992). Progressive myoclonus epilepsies in childhood and adolescence. In: Roger, J., Bureau, M., Dravet, C., Dreifuss, F.E., Wolf, P. and Perret, A. (Eds), *Epileptic Syndromes in Infancy, Childhood and Adolescence, 2nd edn*, John Libbey, London, pp. 381–400.

Roger, J., Bureau, M., Oller Ferrer Vidal, L., Oller-Daurella, L., Saltarelli, A. and Genton, P. (1994). Clinical and electroencephalographic criteria of idiopathic generalized epilepsies. In: Malafosse, A., Genton, P., Hirsch, E., Marescaux, C., Broglin, D. and Bernasconi, R. (Eds), *Idiopathic Generalized Epilepsies: Clinical, Experimental and Genetic Aspects.* John Libbey, London, pp. 7–18.

Salas-Puig, X., Camara da Silva, A.M., Dravet, C. and Roger, J. (1990). L'épilepsie myoclonique juvénile dans la population du Centre Saint Paul. *Epilepsies* **2**, 108–113.

Serratosa, J.M. and Delgado-Escueta, A.V. (1993). Juvenile myoclonic epilepsy. In: Wyllie, E. (Ed.), *The Treatment of Epilepsy. Principles and Practice.* Lea and Febiger, Philadelphia, pp. 552–570.

So, G.M., Thiele, E.A., Sanger, T., Schmid, R. and Riviello, J.J. (1998). Electroencephalogram and clinical focalities in juvenile myoclonic epilepsy. *J Child Neurol* **13**, 541–545.

Sözüer, D.T., Atakli, D., Atay, T., Baybas, S. and Arpaci, B. (1996). Evaluation of various antiepileptic drugs in juvenile myoclonic epilepsy. *Epilepsia* **37** (suppl 4), S77.

Su, Y.H., Izumi, T., Kitsu, M. and Fukuyama, Y. (1993). Seizure threshold in juvenile myoclonic epilepsy with Graves' disease. *Epilepsia* **34**, 488–492.

Topcuoglu, M.A., Saygi, S. and Ciger, A. (1997). Rotatory seizures in juvenile myoclonic epilepsy. *Clin Neurol Neurosurg* **99**, 248–251.

Touchon, J., Besset, A., Billiard, M. and Baldy-Moulinier, M. (1982). Effects of spontaneous and provoked awakening on the frequency of polyspike and wave discharges in 'bilateral massive epileptic myoclonus'. In: Akimoto, H., Kazamatsuri, M., Seino, M. and Ward, M. (Eds), *Advances in Epileptology, Vol. 13.* Raven Press, New York, pp. 269–272.

Tsuboi, T. (1977). *Primary Generalized Epilepsy with Sporadic Myoclonias of Myoclonic Petit Mal Type.* Thieme, Stuttgart.

Wallace, S.J. (1998). Myoclonus and epilepsy in childhood: a review of treatment with valproate, ethosuximide, lamotrigine and zonisamide. *Epilepsy Res* **29**, 147–154.

Wolf, P. (1985) Benign juvenile myoclonic epilepsy. In: Roger, J., Dravet, Ch., Bureau, M., Dreifuss, F.E. and Wolf, P. (Eds), *Epileptic Syndromes in Infancy, Childhood and Adolescence.* John Libbey, London, pp. 242–246.

Wolf, P. (1992a). Juvenile myoclonic epilepsy. In: Roger, J., Bureau, M., Dravet, Ch., Dreifuss, F.E., Perret, A. and Wolf, P. (Eds), *Epileptic Syndromes in Infancy, Childhood and Adolescence, 2nd edn.* John Libbey, London, pp. 313–327.

Wolf, P. (1992b). Juvenile absence epilepsy. In: Roger, J., Bureau, M., Dravet, Ch., Dreifuss, F.E., Perret, A. and Wolf, P. (Eds), *Epileptic Syndromes in Infancy, Childhood and Adolescence, 2nd edn.* John Libbey, London, pp. 307–312.

Wolf, P. (1992c). Epilepsy with grand mal on awakening. In: Roger, J., Bureau, M., Dravet, Ch., Dreifuss, F.E., Perret, A. and Wolf, P. (Eds), *Epileptic Syndromes in Infancy, Childhood and Adolescence, 2nd edn.* John Libbey, London, pp. 329–341.

Juvenile Myoclonic Epilepsy: The Janz Syndrome
Edited by Bettina Schmitz and Thomas Sander
© 2000 Wrightson Biomedical Publishing Ltd

4

Juvenile Myoclonic Epilepsy: A Syndrome Challenging Syndromic Concepts?

PETER WOLF and THOMAS MAYER

Epilepsie-Zentrum Bethel, Bielefeld, Germany

DEFINITION

A syndrome is, according to the definition of the International Classification of Epilepsies and Epileptic Syndromes (ICEES), 'a cluster of signs and symptoms customarily occurring together ... in contradistinction to a disease, a syndrome does not necessarily have a common etiology and prognosis' (Commission on Classification and Terminology of the ILAE, 1989). This sounds very straightforward. However, in epileptology, there is perhaps something more to be said about a syndrome and this 'something more' is contained in the definition of 'idiopathic' epilepsies in which it is stated: '... there is no underlying cause other than a possible hereditary predisposition' – which indicates a possibility of a common etiology. Idiopathic epilepsy syndromes, thus, are candidate epilepsies, candidate diseases. Once a specific gene (or a specific cluster of genes in plurigenetic disorders) is localized, identified and, eventually, its (or their) pathogenic mode of action clarified, there is no reason to maintain the resulting disorder in the class of syndromes: it will have become a disease.

Juvenile myoclonic epilepsy (JME) is one of the well described syndromes of idiopathic generalized epilepsy. Its description in the ICEES reads as follows:

Juvenile myoclonic epilepsy (impulsive petit mal)
Impulsive petit mal appears around puberty and is characterized by seizures with bilateral, single or repetitive, arrhythmic, irregular myoclonic jerks, predominantly in the arms. Jerks may cause some patients to fall suddenly. No disturbance of consciousness is noticeable. The disorder may be inherited, and sex distribution is equal. Often there are GTCS (generalized tonic–clonic seizures) and, less often, infre-

quent absences. The seizures usually occur shortly after awakening and are often precipitated by sleep deprivation. Interictal and ictal EEG have rapid, generalized, often irregular spike-waves and polyspike-waves; there is no close phase correlation between EEG spikes and jerks. Frequently, the patients are photosensitive. Response to appropriate drugs is good.

GENETIC APPROACHES

Certainly, a well delineated clinical syndrome such as this, where an important hereditary component was recognized early, was a good candidate for genetic clarification, and JME indeed became an early object of modern, syndrome-orientated genetic research in epilepsy. In this volume, a comprehensive update of the results of this research is given.

Clinical epileptologists were pleased but not surprised when they heard the first reports about a gene locus having been identified in JME. However, the question remained whether this was where 'the' gene for JME was located, or whether it was perhaps one of multiple genes involved in this disorder.

Initially, for example, it could not be ruled out that this was perhaps the gene locus for photosensitivity, because sensitivity to intermittent light is a hereditary trait which is frequent in JME. Wolf and Goosses (1986) found that no other epilepsy syndrome was as closely related to photosensitivity. Of 115 patients with JME in their study, 30.5% were photosensitive. In females, the rate was still higher (40%), and there were methodological reasons why these figures had to be considered as representing only a minimum. A recent British study has indeed proposed a much higher rate of photosensitivity (Beirne et al., 1998).

However, the euphoria about the first gene locus which was discovered in one of the major epilepsy syndromes made many forget that this only probable and still imprecise locus was merely an indicator. It was not clear what was indicated or what exactly it had to do with JME.

A HOMOGENEOUS SYNDROME?

We have become wiser since then, as it has been realized that less was known than assumed. We have learned that the syndrome cannot be linked in all families to chromosome 6 which indicates that, whatever is located there, is not *the* gene for JME. It was necessary to realize that, unless the variance is explained by gene translocation, JME is probably not genetically homogeneous. It may be that

- various genes produce highly similar phenotypes, or

- the clinical syndrome is caused by an interaction of various genes, or
- the clinical syndrome is less homogeneous than was believed, and we have not been sufficiently attentive to notice the differences.

The geneticists have thrown the ball back into the field of clinical epileptology to look at the syndrome again. Is it one clinical syndrome or, as with the absence epilepsies, a group of syndromes which are very similar but distinguishable? Or is there a homogeneous core syndrome with some modifiers, traits which may be present or absent? In the latter case, we still could hope to find a major JME gene which interacts with modifier genes.

REFLEX EPILEPTIC TRAITS IN JME

When we talk about possible accessory traits, or of subgroups in JME, an obvious distinction would be that of photosensitive versus non-photosensitive patients. A study is still awaited which makes this differentiation. It was not made in the early genetic investigations where, in view of its high frequency, photosensitivity certainly was present in a substantial part of the families on which the chromosome 6p localization was based, but surely not in all. In this respect, the investigated population cannot have been homogeneous. However, there are other possibilities.

Some years ago, the group of Shizuoka (Inoue *et al.*, 1994) drew attention to another trait, which is discussed in this volume by Inoue (Chapter 7). They were able to collect and study a relatively large series of patients with what was usually called seizures by decision-making, by calculation, by complex cognitive tasks or by chess and card games. The authors deserve credit to have discovered that, in these cases, it was typically a complex interaction of thinking with a manual task that precipitated seizures. Their term 'praxis-induced seizures' very well describes this combined mental and manual trigger of seizures. Several of their patients had seizures when they did calculations with the traditional Japanese abacus, the 'soroban'. This activity is a perfect example of praxis in the sense of cognitive involvement combined with a differentiated manual task, and the usually rapid performance enhances the stimulus.

The Shizuoka group deserves special credit for looking more closely at the clinical syndromes of these patients, and finding that, indeed, JME seemed to be the syndrome most closely linked with praxis induction.

JME AND READING EPILEPSY

In recent years there have been several reports of a co-occurrence of JME with primary reading epilepsy (PRE). This is a syndrome which belongs to the group of idiopathic localization-related epilepsies, with a specific hereditary background, and where all seizures are precipitated by reading. Radhakrishnan *et al.* (1995) diagnosed a combination with JME in four of their 20 patients with PRE, and the authors have observed it in an additional three cases (Mayer and Wolf, 1997). They all had in common that the features of the two syndromes did not become mixed. Reading provoked small, lightening-like lingual and perioral myocloni which are the characteristic feature of PRE, whereas the bilateral jerks of the upper limbs typical for JME were never precipitated by reading but occurred spontaneously, mostly in the morning hours and after sleep deprivation. In most of these patients, the features of the two syndromes had a different age of onset.

Can one person have two epilepsies? Perhaps, as an extreme hazard this may happen. But what is the significance of multiple observations of co-occurrence of two well defined particular syndromes? They cannot be due to chance. We are used to viewing the border between generalized and localization-related epilepsies as a deep gulf. Is that correct? What is it that can relate the two syndromes across this gulf? Here is indeed a challenge to our syndromic concepts. Are these two plurigenetic hereditary syndromes which share one gene but whose other genes differ? Is the difference between focal and generalized epilepsy gradual rather than fundamental? Is this dichotomy, in idiopathic epilepsies, just a question of bilateral symmetric versus unilateral or strongly asymmetric regional gene expression? These are fascinating questions which are not easy to answer.

RECENT FINDINGS

Intrigued by the observations of a combination of PRE and JME, one of the authors (TM) has since 1994 started regularly to question all new patients he sees in the outpatient clinic of the authors' centre about the precipitation of seizures or perioral/lingual myoclonias by reading. Of about 600 patients, in 17 who believed they had experienced such phenomena this report could be confirmed by prolonged EEG–video recordings including reading tests in German and English. None of them had primary reading epilepsy, i.e. seizures exclusively precipitated by reading. This indicates that the perioral reflex-myoclonias which are the hallmark of PRE may occur, as a trait, in about 3% of all patients with epilepsy.

In addition to these 17 ambulatory patients with what has been called 'secondary reading epilepsy' (Bickford *et al.*, 1956) who were detected by systematic questioning, another seven patients were identified, in the same period, on the wards of the Epilepsy Centre Bethel, Hospital Mara, in consequence of a generally increased awareness of this diagnosis or trait (Table 1).

Table 1. Perioral myocloni precipitated by talking and reading (PMPTR).

Patients with PMPTR	24
Syndrome diagnoses:	
Juvenile myoclonic epilepsy	12
Epilepsy with GM on awaking	2
Symptomatic/cryptogenic focal epilepsy	10

Note: Sample comprised 17 of approximately 600 newly admitted ambulatory patients between 1994 and 1998 (3%) and seven inpatients (not systematically collected).
GM: grand mal.

A preliminary observation of these 24 patients as a group is that their perioral myoclonias seem to be precipitated by talking as much as or even more than by reading. This is somewhat different from PRE where talking provoked myocloni in only about 27% of the published cases (Wolf, 1992). We will therefore refer to the trait as 'perioral myoclonias precipitated by talking and reading' (PMPTR).

Of the 24 patients with PMPTR, the syndrome diagnosis was JME in 12, and epilepsy with grand mal on awakening in another two. Somewhat surprisingly, the remaining 10 suffered from symptomatic or cryptogenic focal epilepsy. Thus, in addition to photosensitivity and precipitation by praxis, still another, third reflex epileptic trait seems to be related to Janz syndrome.

To obtain a clearer idea of the relevance of the two more recently identified traits, precipitation by praxis and by talking/reading, in JME, the authors are conducting a questionnaire survey of all ambulatory patients with this diagnosis who are in long-term treatment with either author (Table 2).

The questionnaire was sent to 86 patients with a diagnosis of JME, and 62 (72%) responded. Discounting nonspecific precipitating mechanisms such as sleep withdrawal, 'stress', alcohol, or drug non-compliance, 31 of these patients (i.e. one half) answered 'yes' to questions about specific precipitating stimuli. Seven of these positive responses concerned seizure precipitation by intermittent light stimuli. Nineteen responses referred to 'praxis' and

Table 2. Questionnaire on specific seizure precipitation in JME.

Ambulatory JME patients	86
Responses	62 (72%)
Self-reports of specific precipitation	31 (50%)
Praxis	19 (31%)
Talking/reading	14 (23%)
Intermittent lights	7 (11%)

JME: juvenile myoclonic epilepsy.

comprised stimuli such as writing (7), decision-making (4), computer tasks and video games (6), calculations (6), thinking (8), and playing the piano (1).

Fourteen patients reported perioral myoclonias precipitated by talking (delivering a speech in five), and eight in addition by reading.

Nine patients reported precipitation by both praxis and talking/reading. These are very preliminary findings which now will be subject to detailed investigations. But whatever the final figures may be, it seems safe to assume that reflex epileptic traits of at least three different types are quite common in this syndrome, in which until recently we believed nonspecific stimuli, such as sleep withdrawal, to be much more important.

Video documentation confirmed, in a number of these patients from the authors' investigation with JME, the following findings:

- perioral myoclonias precipitated by both reading and talking
- minimal orolingual myoclonias precipitated by reading and talking, and jerks of the right hand during writing (spontaneous or to dictation) in one patient
- manual jerks precipitated by playing the piano in another.

GENERALIZED, LOCALIZATION-RELATED AND REGIONAL EPILEPTIC ACTIVITY

What all these patients have in common is that some local motor activity on which the patient's attention is focused provokes local myoclonic phenomena or, as Bickford put it in his first description of reading epilepsy, that 'proprioceptive bombardment' results in 'reflex firing through the same motor segment' (Bickford *et al.*, 1956). The most surprising aspect is of course that these minimal, truly partial motor seizures happen in a condition which is considered a 'generalized' epilepsy syndrome. Furthermore, the reflex-like phenomena observed look a good deal different from the bilateral brachial jerks which we are used to thinking of as the typical seizure of Janz syndrome, and which do occur in the same patients.

Perhaps this is the right place to remember that it is a mere convention to call the bilateral motor manifestations in JME 'generalized' merely because the concomitant EEG will show polyspike-waves over the entire cortex. The seizure semiology, however, remains restricted to a rather circumscribed area.

At the Bethel-Cleveland Symposium of 1993 (Wolf, 1994), many of the contributions and discussions were concerned with the relation of the widespread bilateral discharges, which by convention are today called 'generalized', to the – bilateral or unilateral – regional expression of clinical symptoms. This discussion needs perhaps to be pursued. One of the open questions in this respect is, in photosensitive JME patients, by what intermediaries does the occipital cortical input of intermittent lights produce myoclonic jerks of the extremities. Still, these are bilateral and roughly symmetric. The observations reported above add even more intriguing questions about direct, reflex-like sensorimotor interactions on a much more localized level, within the realm of a 'generalized' syndrome.

These observations seem to indicate that the distinction between focal and generalized epileptic phenomena may be sharper in the minds of epileptologists than in reality. It may to some extent be artificial. The closer we look at the prototype of an idiopathic generalized epilepsy syndrome, JME or Janz syndrome, the more we have to realize, so it seems, that it is indeed a syndrome which challenges our syndromic concepts.

REFERENCES

Beirne, M., Acomb, B. and Appleton, R. (1998). Photosensitivity in juvenile myoclonic epilepsy. *Seizure* **7**, 427.

Bickford, R.G., Whelan, J.L., Klass, D.W. and Corbin, K.B (1956). Reading epilepsy: clinical and electroencephalographic studies of a new syndrome. *Trans Am Neurol Assoc* **81**, 100–102.

Commission on Classification and Terminology of the International League Against Epilepsy (1989). Proposal for revised classification of epilepsies and epileptic syndromes. *Epilepsia* **30**, 389–399.

Inoue, Y., Seino, M., Kubota, H., Yamakaku, K., Tanaka, M. and Yagi, K. (1994). Epilepsy with praxis-induced seizures. In: Wolf, P. (Ed.), *Epileptic Seizures and Syndromes*. John Libbey, London, pp. 81–92.

Mayer, T. and Wolf, P. (1997). Reading epilepsy: related to juvenile myoclonic epilepsy? *Epilepsia* **38** (suppl. 3), 18–19.

Radhakrishnan, K., Silbert, L. and Klass, D.W. (1995). Reading epilepsy. An appraisal of 20 patients diagnosed at the Mayo Clinic, Rochester, Minnesota, between 1949 and 1989, and delineation of the epileptic syndrome. *Brain* **118**, 75–89.

Wolf, P. and Goosses, R. (1986). Relation of photosensitivity to epileptic syndromes. *J Neurol Neurosurg Psychiatry* **49**, 1386–1391.

Wolf, P. (1992). Reading epilepsy. In: Roger, J., Bureau, M., Dravet, C., Dreifuss, F.E., Perret, A. and Wolf, P. (Eds), *Epileptic Syndromes in Infancy, Childhood and Adolescence*. John Libbey, London, pp. 281–298.

Wolf, P. (Ed.) (1994). *Epileptic Seizures and Syndromes*. John Libbey, London.

Juvenile Myoclonic Epilepsy: The Janz Syndrome
Edited by Bettina Schmitz and Thomas Sander
© 2000 Wrightson Biomedical Publishing Ltd

5

The EEG in Juvenile Myoclonic Epilepsy

STEPHAN WALTZ

Neuropaediatric Department, University of Kiel, Kiel, Germany

INTRODUCTION

In their original work on juvenile myoclonic epilepsy (JME), Janz and Christian in 1957 gave a detailed description of the characteristic electroencephalographic features. Janz (1969) was the first to distinguish the different syndromes of idiopathic generalized epilepsy as recognized today by the International Classification of the International League Against Epilepsy. Janz (1969) attached classical 3/s spikes and waves to pyknoleptic absences or childhood absence epilepsy, the faster 4–6/s spike wave variant to juvenile absence epilepsy, and polyspikes and waves to JME. Since then, polyspikes and waves have been regarded as the typical electroencephalographic correlate of JME and a considerable number of studies concerning the electroencephalogram (EEG) in JME have been performed. In this chapter, current knowledge about EEG findings in JME will be summarized.

SPIKES AND WAVES

Spikes and waves of any kind are found in 44–81% (Canevini *et al.*, 1992; Murthy *et al.*, 1998; Panayiotopoulos *et al.*, 1994; Pedersen and Petersen, 1998; Tsuboi, 1977) of patients with JME. However, repeated recordings and recordings after sleep deprivation can be necessary to register typical findings (Janz and Christian, 1957; Tsuboi, 1977; Genton *et al.*, 1995; Murthy *et al.*, 1998). Pantazis (1989) found generalized paroxysmal activity (including photosensitivity) in 84% of patients with three or fewer EEG recordings. This rate increased up to 96% in patients with four to eight recordings and remained unchanged in those with more than eight recordings. Duration of

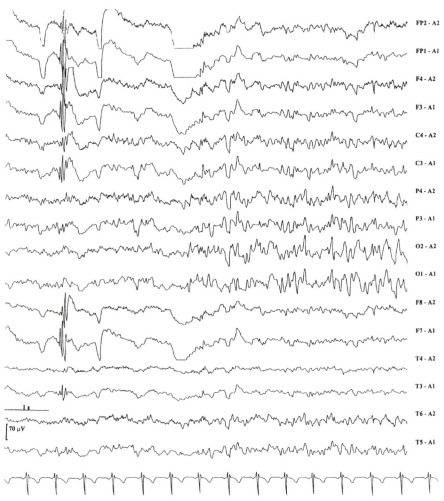

Figure 1. Interictal bilateral single polyspike-wave complex with incomplete generalization.

spike-wave discharges was found to be 0.5–20.0 s (mean 6.8 seconds) by Panayiotopoulos *et al.* (1994).

In interictal discharges, single polyspike-wave complexes may be seen (Figure 1), which sometimes are not completely generalized, but confined to the frontal or central region (Figure 2). Isolated spikes or polyspikes with incomplete generalization may eventually suggest focal discharges. Short trains of irregular spikes and waves (Figure 3) or regular monospikes and waves may also be found (Figure 4). Spike-wave discharges in JME were

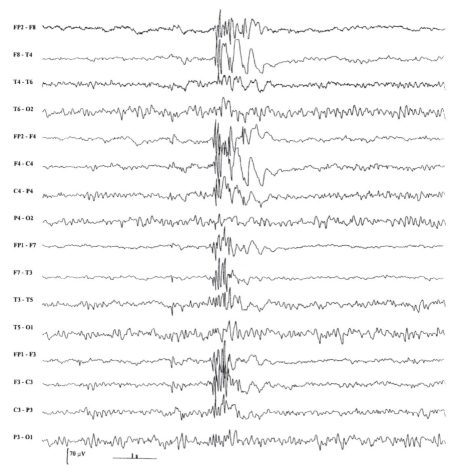

Figure 2. Interictal polyspike-wave complex followed by two slow waves, predominantly over the frontal regions.

described as being often 'fragmented' by Panayiotopoulos and co-workers (Panayiotopoulos *et al.*, 1989, 1994). In an attempt to quantify this impression, Murthy *et al.* (1998) found fragmented discharges in 16% of JME patients.

POLYSPIKES AND WAVES

Janz and Christian in 1957 described in detail the polyspike-wave complex, which they considered to be pathognomonic for JME. They pointed out that usually 5–20 spikes with a frequency of 12–15 Hz precede the slow wave.

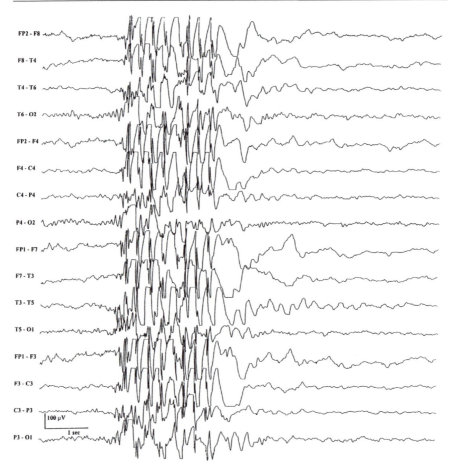

Figure 3. Generalized rapid irregular spikes and waves with initial polyspikes.

Table 1. Juvenile myoclonic epilepsy: spikes and waves.

Authors	N	2.5–3.5/s sw (%)	4–6/s sw (%)	Polysw (%)
Tsuboi (1977)	381	11	22	26
Asconapé and Penry (1984)	12	nr	nr	58
Delgado-Escueta & Enrile-Bacsal (1984)	43	nr	——100,——	
Clement and Wallace (1988)	10	——80——		60
Pantazis (1989)	181	55	52	49
Canevini et al. (1992)	35	——60——		37
Genton et al. (1994)	82	16	82	45
Pedersen and Petersen (1998)	36	0	22	22
Bittermann and Steinhoff (1998)	30	——57——		43

nr: not reported.

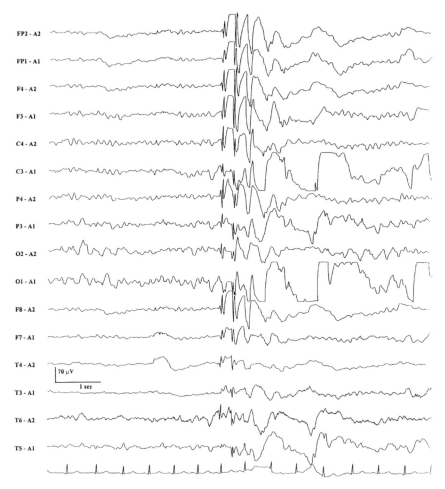

Figure 4. Interictal generalized 3.5–4/s monospikes and waves.

Amplitudes of the spikes could reach 150–300 μV. The frequency of the slow waves was found to be 3–5 Hz; amplitudes were usually 200–350 μV. In later studies, polyspikes and waves were found in 22–60% of JME patients (Table 1). The first, largest and the only comparative study was performed by Tsuboi (1977). In a retrospective study of 381 JME patients and 466 patients with other types of epilepsy, he found polyspikes and waves more often in JME than in other epileptic syndromes, although only in a minority (26%) of JME patients. Polyspikes and waves were also found in other syndromes of idiopathic generalized epilepsy as well as in a small number of patients with focal epilepsy. Moreover, he showed that other types of spikes and waves, such as 3/s SW (11%), 4–6/s SW (21.5%) may also be found in JME. Later statistical analysis of interictal discharges failed to confirm that polyspikes and waves are more common in JME than other types of spikes and waves (Table 1). Most authors found 3/s sw and/or 4–6/s SW more often than polyspikes and waves (Clement and Wallace, 1988; Pantazis, 1989; Genton et al., 1994; Bittermann and Steinhoff, 1998). All studies were retrospective and most patients were treated with antiepileptic drugs at the time of investigation. Most epileptologists will agree that polyspikes and waves are a characteristic finding in JME. However, there is no evidence that polyspikes and waves are a finding specific for JME nor can it be considered mandatory for diagnosis.

ICTAL DISCHARGES

Janz and Christian (1957) registered myoclonic seizures in 16 patients and noticed that no clinically manifest impulsive petit mal occurs without polyspikes and waves. They found that in ictal discharges, the polyspike-wave complex is often preceded by some irregular 2–3/s slow waves, which may be interrupted by isolated spikes or double-spikes. Duration of ictal discharges was found to be 2–20 seconds, often longer than the clinically apparent myoclonic jerks (Janz and Christian, 1957). The number of spikes appeared to correlate with the intensity, but not with the duration of the myoclonic jerks. Onset of discharges were often in the frontal or central region with consecutive spread to the parietal, temporal and occipital regions. Since then only little information on ictal discharges has been collected (Delgado-Escueta and Enrile-Bacsal, 1984; Waltz et al., 1990; Oguni et al., 1994). In a comparative study, polyspikes and waves occurred in all myoclonic seizures, whereas this was the case in 26% of absence seizures (Waltz et al., 1990). Delgado-Escueta and Enrile-Bacsal (1984) found repetitive medium-high amplitude 10–16 Hz spikes during generalized myoclonic jerks in eight patients. These discharges were sometimes preceded by diffuse irregular 2–5 Hz spike-wave complexes and followed by irregular high amplitude 1–3 Hz slow waves. Oguni et al. (1994) found that in myoclonic seizures occurring repeatedly, each jerk corresponded to a burst of generalized spikes and waves or polyspikes and waves at 3–5 Hz, which lasted one to two seconds and rarely as long as four seconds. Interictal discharges appeared to be of smaller amplitude than ictal discharges.

HYPERVENTILATION

Hyperventilation has been reported to provoke spikes and waves in 25–100% (Tsuboi, 1977; Pantazis, 1989; Canevini et al., 1992; Oguni et al., 1994;

Table 2. Juvenile myoclonic epilepsy: effect of hyperventilation.

Authors	N	Provocation of EEG discharges by hyperventilation	
		n	%
Tsuboi (1977)	381	243	64
Pantazis (1989)	181	124	69
Canevini et al. (1992)	60	15	25
Oguni et al. (1994)	5	5	100
Panayiotopoulos et al. (1994)	66	66	100
Pedersen and Petersen (1998)	36	9	25
Total	729	462	63

Panayiotopoulos et al., 1994; Pedersen and Petersen, 1998) of patients with JME (Table 2). Janz and Christian (1957) felt that hyperventilation may not be as effective as in absences. A comparative study has not yet been performed.

SLEEP AND SLEEP DEPRIVATION

Janz and Christian (1957) emphasized that sleep deprivation is the most powerful tool for provoking seizures and spikes and waves in patients with JME. Seizure provocation after sleep deprivation has been confirmed by many investigators (Asconapé and Penry, 1984; Delgado-Escueta and Enrile-Bacsal, 1984; Panayiotopoulos et al., 1994; Bittermann and Steinhoff, 1998; Pedersen and Petersen, 1998). Most investigators emphasize the importance of an EEG recording after sleep deprivation, in case the routine recording is normal. A proper electroencephalographic investigation, however, has not been performed.

Gigli et al., (1991) performed a nocturnal polysomnographic study in an untreated JME patient who showed eye closure sensitivity but no photosensitivity. The rate of polyspikes and waves was high before sleep onset, increased during spontaneous nocturnal awakenings and became maximal during final morning awakening. Discharges were suppressed during rapid eye movement (REM) sleep. During non-REM sleep, discharges were maximal during stages III and IV.

PHOTOSENSITIVITY

A photoparoxysmal response to intermittent light stimulation is a characteristic EEG finding in patients with JME. Photosensitivity is a genetically transmitted EEG trait closely associated with epilepsy (Waltz et al., 1992). It is genetically and pathophysiologically different from spikes and waves at

Table 3. Juvenile myoclonic epilepsy: photosensitivity.

Authors	N	Photosensitive	
		n	%
Covanis et al. (1982)	45	22	49
Asconapé and Penry (1984)	12	4	33
Wolf and Goosses (1986)	121	37	31
Salas-Puig et al. (1988)	24	4	20
Clement and Wallace (1988)	10	4	40
Obeid and Panayiotopoulos (1988)	50	15	30
Oguni and Fukuyama (1988)	14	8	57
Waltz et al. (1990)	181	69	38
Panayiotopoulos et al. (1994)	66	18	27
Aliberti et al. (1994)	22	13	59
Genton et al. (1994)	82	28	33
Atakli et al. (1998)	76	20	26
Bittermann and Steinhoff (1998)	30	6	20
Total	709	244	34

rest or hyperventilation (Doose and Waltz, 1993). Photosensitivity has been found in 20–57% (mean 34%) of patients with JME (Table 3). All figures given in the literature have probably to be considered as a minimum estimate for two reasons. First, most patients have been treated with antiepileptic drugs, mostly with valproate, which may abolish the photoparoxysmal response. Secondly, most studies have been performed mainly in adults

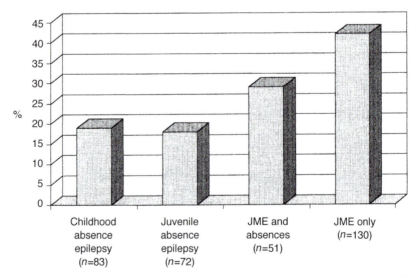

Figure 5. Rate of photosensitivity depending on the occurrence of myoclonic seizures in syndromes of generalized epilepsy (adapted from Waltz et al., 1990).

(Wolf, 1992). Those from paediatric departments with younger patients (Clement and Wallace, 1988; Oguni and Fukuyama, 1988) tend to find higher rates of photosensitivity.

Within the idiopathic generalized epilepsies, photosensitivity appears to be closely correlated with JME. Wolf and Goosses (1986) found photosensitivity more often in JME than in all other epileptic syndromes. In an investigation of 337 patients with idiopathic generalized epilepsy, patients with JME without absences showed the trait in 42%. Patients with either childhood absence epilepsy or juvenile absence epilepsy displayed photosensitivity in 19% and 18% respectively. Patients with both JME and absences showed an intermediate rate of 29% (Figure 5). Although photosensitivity is a frequent finding

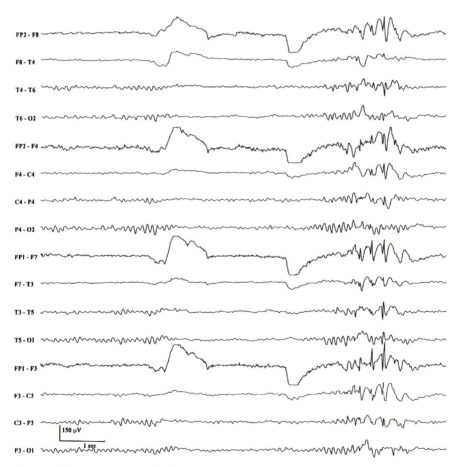

Figure 6. Eye closure sensitivity: incompletely generalized and slightly asymmetric spikes and waves induced by eye closure.

Table 4. Juvenile myoclonic epilepsy: eye closure sensitivity.

Authors	N	Eye closure sensitivity	
		n	%
Goosses (1984)	121	26	21
Obeid and Panayiotopoulos (1988)	50	3	6
Canevini *et al.* (1992)	60	5	8
Panayiotopoulos *et al.* (1994)	66	2	14
Murthy *et al.* (1998)	131	6	5
Total	376	42	11

in JME, it also may occur in all other epileptic syndromes (Wolf and Goosses, 1986; Waltz, 1994) as well as in healthy subjects (Doose and Waltz, 1993).

EYE CLOSURE SENSITIVITY

Eye closure sensitivity (Table 4) is defined by the reproducible provocation of spikes and waves within two seconds after eye closure (Figure 6). It is closely related to photosensitivity and has to be distinguished from other eye-closed related discharges as fixation-off sensitivity. Janz and Christian (1957) and later Asconapé and Penry (1984) reported JME patients who had myoclonic jerks provoked by eye closure. Canevini *et al.* (1992) suggested that the combination of sleep deprivation or awakening and eye closure may be an important seizure-triggering factor.

Electroencephalographic eye closure sensitivity was found in 5–20% of patients with JME (Goosses, 1984; Obeid and Panayiotopoulos, 1988; Canevini *et al.*, 1992; Panayiotopoulos *et al.*, 1994; Murthy *et al.*, 1998). The rate of eye closure sensitivity may depend on the number of EEG recordings which have been evaluated, as figures are high in studies evaluating a larger number of recordings (Goosses, 1984 (20%); Panayiotopoulos *et al.*, 1994 (14%)) whereas the lowest figure (5%) is found in the study of Murthy *et al.* (1998) who evaluated the initial EEG recording only.

FOCAL FINDINGS

There have been a considerable number of reports on focal EEG abnormalities in JME in recent years (Table 5). Focal abnormalities or 'asymmetries' (Obeid and Panayiotopoulos, 1988; Lancmann *et al.*, 1994) have been reported in 8–55% of patients (mean 21%; Table 3). Focal findings may consist of voltage asymmetries, unilateral onset of generalized discharges, focal slowing or focal spikes (Aliberti *et al.*, 1994; Lancmann *et al.*, 1994;

Table 5. Juvenile myoclonic epilepsy: focal EEG abnormalities.

Authors	N	Focal abnormalities	
		n	%
Asconapé and Penry (1984)	12	1	8
Obeid and Panayiotopoulos (1988)[a]	50	17	34
Pantazis (1989)	181	21	12
Panayiotopoulos et al. (1994)	66	20	30
Aliberti et al. (1994)	22	12	55
Lancmann et al. (1994)[b]	85	26	31
Genton et al. (1994)	82	13	16
Murthy et al. (1998)	131	27	21
Atakli et al. (1998)	76	15	20
Pedersen and Petersen (1998)	36	5	14
Bittermann and Steinhoff (1998)	30	5	17
Total	771	162	21

[a]including asymmetries.
[b]'significant EEG asymmetries'.

Murthy et al., 1998). The most common finding is voltage asymmetry (Aliberti et al., 1994; Murthy et al., 1998). Only in a minority of cases were these changes consistent through all recordings or consistently unilateral. Continuous focal slowing appears to be rare (Aliberti et al., 1994). The significance of such focal findings remains to be established. Lancmann and co-workers (1994) found that patients with EEG asymmetries do not differ clinically from those without asymmetries. However, delay in diagnosis was greater in patients with asymmetries.

BACKGROUND ACTIVITY

Most investigators found background activity in JME undisturbed. Slowing of background activity was found in 0% (Asconapé and Penry, 1984; Delgado-Escueta and Enrile-Bacsal, 1984; Canevini et al., 1992), 10% (Janz and Christian, 1957; Clement and Wallace, 1988) and 42% (Panayiotopoulos et al., 1994). Janz and Christian in 1957 noticed that a very regular, high-voltage alpha EEG was typically found in JME. Tsuboi (1977) found 'high-voltage alpha-activity' significantly more often in patients with JME than in controls. Such a regular alpha-EEG was described by Dieker (1967). He called it monotonous alpha-EEG and reported an autosomal-dominant transmission of this normal EEG trait. Examples of monotonous alpha-EEG in patients with JME can be found in illustrations provided by Janz and Christian (1957), Janz (1969) and Delgado-Escueta and Enrile-Bacsal (1984).

Doose and co-workers (1995) conducted a family study in a paediatric population and found this specific kind of alpha-activity significantly more

often in parents of children with idiopathic generalized epilepsy (IGE) and
spikes and waves on the EEG than in parents of children with focal epilepsy
or healthy controls. By contrast, background activity lacking alpha waves (i.e.
beta-EEG, low voltage-EEG) were found significantly more often in the
latter groups. It may therefore be possible that this physiological EEG trait
may indicate an increased genetic risk for IGE with spikes and waves.

JUVENILE MYOCLONIC EPILEPSY WITH ABSENCES

Approximately one-third of patients with JME may also have absences (Janz
and Waltz, 1995). These absences are often short with only mild impairment
of consciousness and therefore may only be diagnosed during EEG recording (Panayiotopoulos et al., 1989). Pantazis (1989) found no difference
between JME patients with absences and those without absences regarding
overall rate of spikes and waves, activating effect of hyperventilation and
rates of different types of spikes and waves. By contrast, patients with JME
and absences showed polyspikes and waves significantly more often than
patients with absences only (Table 6; Waltz et al., 1993). Photosensitivity was
found less often in JME patients with additional absences (29%) than in JME
patients without absences (42%) (see Figure 5).

DIAGNOSTIC VALUE OF THE EEG

Many recent reports on JME emphasize that JME still is an underdiagnosed
syndrome (Panayiotopoulos et al., 1991; Salas Puig et al., 1994; Atakli et al.,
1998; Bittermann and Steinhoff, 1998; Murthy et al., 1998). Misinterpretation
of the EEG has been reported to contribute to the diagnostic delay in
21–75% of misdiagnosed cases (Atakli et al., 1998; Murthy et al., 1998). EEG
recordings were interpreted either as indicative of focal epilepsy or as consistent with other syndromes of idiopathic generalized epilepsy. In some cases
the finding of 3–3.5/s SW was thought to indicate absence epilepsy (Murthy
et al., 1998). The value of the initial EEG recording has been addressed by
three investigators (Tsuboi, 1977; Genton et al., 1995; Murthy et al., 1998).
They found diagnostic EEG changes in 54–81% of patients. Genton et al.
(1995) reported 'misleading changes', mainly focal findings in 20% of recordings. All authors stressed the importance of repeated EEG recordings when
the diagnosis is not clear and pointed out that EEG recording after sleep
deprivation is the most important and most powerful diagnostic procedure.
Pantazis (1989) showed that in some patients four to eight recordings including hyperventilation and photic stimulation may be necessary to register
generalized paroxysmal activity.

Table 6. Juvenile myoclonic epilepsy with absences.

	N	2.5–3.5/s sw (%)	4–6/s sw (%)	Polysw (%)
Childhood absence epilepsy	72	*78	**64	47
Juvenile absence epilepsy	54	*44	76	33
Total absence epilepsies	126	63	69	***41
JME with absences	19	63	**90	***68

*p <0.001; **p <0.01; ***p <0.05.
Source: Adapted from Waltz et al., 1993.

Misinterpretation of EEG findings in patients with JME may be minimized when the investigator is aware that normal recordings and some sort of focal EEG findings can be registered in a considerable number of patients with JME. Likewise, registration of absences is no argument against a diagnosis of JME. The available literature does not support the assumption of an inter-ictal EEG marker specific for JME. The EEG as a diagnostic tool may therefore support a diagnosis of idiopathic generalized epilepsy and may show features *suggestive* of JME. Definite diagnosis of the specific syndrome, however, will rely on careful evaluation of the clinical history unless an ictal recording is available.

REFERENCES

Aliberti V., Grünwald R.A., Panayiotopoulos, C.P. and Chroni, E. (1994). Focal electroencephalographic abnormalities in juvenile myoclonic epilepsy. *Epilepsia* **35**, 297–301.

Asconapé, J. and Penry J.K. (1984). Some clinical and EEG aspects of benign juvenile myoclonic epilepsy. *Epilepsia* **25**, 108–114.

Atakli, D., Sözüer, D., Atay, T., Baybas, S. and Arpaci, B. (1998). Misdiagnosis and treatment in juvenile myoclonic epilepsy. *Seizure* **7**, 63–66.

Bittermann, H.J. and Steinhoff, B.J. (1998). Juvenile myoclonic epilepsy (Janz syndrome). A well-known epilepsy syndrome? *Nervenarzt* **69**, 127–130.

Canevini, M.P., Mai, R., Di Marco, C. *et al.* (1992). Juvenile myoclonic epilepsy of Janz: clinical observations in 60 patients. *Seizure* **1**, 291–298.

Clement, M.J. and Wallace, S.J. (1988). Juvenile myoclonic epilepsy. *Arch Dis Child* **63**, 1049–1953.

Covanis, A., Gupta, A.K. and Jeavons, P.M. (1982). Sodium valproate: monotherapy and polytherapy. *Epilepsia* **23**, 693–720.

Delgado-Escueta, A.V. and Enrile-Bacsal, F. (1984). Juvenile myoclonic epilepsy of Janz. *Neurology* **34**, 285–294.

Dieker, H. (1967). Studies on the genetics of particularly regular high alpha-waves in human EEG. *Humangenetik* **4**, 189–216.

Doose, H. and Waltz, S. (1993). Photosensitivity: genetics and clinical significance. *Neuropediatrics* **24**, 250–255.

Doose, H., Castiglione, E. and Waltz, S. (1995). Parental generalized EEG alpha activity predisposes to spike wave discharges in offspring. *Hum Genet* **96**, 695–704.

Genton, P., Salas Puig, X., Tunon, A., Lahoz, C.H., del Socorra, M. and Sanchez, G. (1994). Juvenile myoclonic epilepsy and related syndromes: clinical and neurophysiological aspects. In: Malafosse, A., Genton, P., Hirsch, E., Marescaux, C., Broglin, D. and Bernasconi, R. (Eds), *Idiopathic Generalized Epilepsies*. John Libbey, London, pp. 253–265.

Genton, P., Gonzalez Sanchez, M.S., Saltarelli, A., Bureau, M., Dravet, C. and Roger, J. (1995). Misleading aspects of the standard electroencephalogram in juvenile myoclonic epilepsy: a retrospective study of 56 consecutive cases. *Neurophysiol Clin* **25**, 283–290.

Gigli, G.L., Calia, E., Luciani, L. *et al.* (1991). Eye closure sensitivity without photosensitivity in juvenile myoclonic epilepsy: polysomnographic study of electroencephalographic epileptiform discharge rates. *Epilepsia* **32**, 677–683.

Goosses, R. (1984). *Die Beziehung der Fotosensibilität zu den verschiedenen epileptischen Syndromen* [Thesis]. Freie Universität, Berlin.

Janz, D. (1969). *Die Epilepsien*. Thieme, Stuttgart.

Janz, D. and Christian, W. (1957). Impulsiv-Petit mal. *Dtsch Z Nervenheilk.* **176**, 346–386.

Janz, D. and Waltz, S. (1995). Juvenile myoclonic epilepsy with absences. In: Duncan, J.S., Panayiotopoulos, C.P. (Eds), *Typical Absences and Related Epileptic Syndromes*. London, Churchill, pp. 174–183.

Lancmann, M.E., Asconapé, J.J. and Penry, J.K. (1994). Clinical and EEG asymmetries in juvenile myoclonic epilepsy. *Epilepsia* **35**, 302–306.

Murthy, J.M., Rao, C.M. and Meena, A.K. (1998). Clinical observations of juvenile myoclonic epilepsy in 131 patients: a study in South India. *Seizure* **7**, 43–47.

Obeid, T. and Panayiotopoulos, C.P. (1988). Juvenile myoclonic epilepsy: a study in Saudi Arabia. *Epilepsia* **29**, 280–282.

Oguni, H. and Fukuyama, Y. (1988). Clinical and electroencephalographical study of the patients with juvenile myoclonic epilepsy. *J Jpn Epilepsy Soc* **6**, 39–46.

Oguni, H., Mukahira, K., Oguni, M. *et al.* (1994). Video-polygraphic analysis of myoclonic seizures in juvenile myoclonic epilepsy. *Epilepsia* **35**, 307–316.

Panayiotopoulos, C.P., Obeid, T. and Waheed, G. (1989). Absences in juvenile myoclonic epilepsy: a clinical and video-electroencephalographic study. *Ann Neurol* **25**, 391–397.

Panayiotopoulos, C.P., Tahan, A.R. and Obeid, T. (1991). Juvenile myoclonic epilepsy: factors of error involved in the diagnosis and treatment. *Epilepsia* **32**, 672–676.

Panayiotopoulos, C.P., Obeid, T. and Tahan, A.R. (1994). Juvenile myoclonic epilepsy: a 5-year prospective study. *Epilepsia* **35**, 285–296.

Pantazis, G. (1989). *Elektroencephalographische Befunde bei der Epilepsie mit Impulsiv-Petit mal* [Thesis]. Freie Universität, Berlin.

Pedersen, S.B. and Petersen, K.A. (1998). Juvenile myoclonic epilepsy: clinical and EEG features. *Acta Neurol Scand* **97**, 160–163.

Salas Puig, J., Gonzalez, C., Tunon, A., Macarron, J., Lahoz, C.H. and Parkas, A. (1988). Epilepsia mioclonica juvenil: aspectos electroclinicos. *Boll Lega It Epil* **62/63**, 199–201.

Salas Puig, J., Tunon, A., Vidal, J.A., Mateos, V., Guisasola, L.M. and Lahoz, C.H. (1994). Janz's juvenile myoclonic epilepsy: a little known frequent syndrome. A study of 85 patients. *Med Clin* **103**, 684–689.

Tsuboi, T. (1977). Primary generalized epilepsy with sporadic myoclonias of myoclonic petit mal type [Thesis]. Stuttgart, Germany.

Waltz, S. (1994). Photosensitivity and epilepsy: a genetic approach. In: Malafosse, A., Genton, P., Hirsch, E., Marescaux, C., Broglin, D. and Bernasconi, R. (Eds), *Idiopathic Generalized Epilepsies*. John Libbey, London, p. 317–328.

Waltz, S., Beck-Mannagetta, G. and Janz, D. (1990). Are there syndrome-related genetically determined spikes and wave patterns? A comparison between syndromes of idiopathic generalized epilepsies. *Epilepsia* **31**, 819.

Waltz, S., Christen, H.-J. and Doose, H. (1992). The different patterns of the photoparoxysmal response. *Electroenceph Clin Neurophysiol* **83**, 138–145.

Waltz, S., Beck-Mannagetta, G. and Janz, D. (1993). Zum Stellenwert des EEG in Diagnose und Differentialdiagnose der idiopathischen generalisierten Epilepsien. *Z. EEG-EMG* **24**, 187.

Wolf, P. (1992). Juvenile myoclonic epilepsy. In: Roger, J., Bureau, M., Dravet, C., Dreifuss, F.E., Perret, A. and Wolf, P. (Eds), *Epileptic Syndromes in Infancy, Childhood and Adolescence*. John Libbey, London, pp. 313–327.

Wolf, P. and Goosses, R. (1986). Relation of photosensitivity to epileptic syndromes. *J Neurol Neurosurg Psychiatry* **49**, 1386–1391.

Juvenile Myoclonic Epilepsy: The Janz Syndrome
Edited by Bettina Schmitz and Thomas Sander
© 2000 Wrightson Biomedical Publishing Ltd

6

Pathophysiology of Myoclonus in Janz Syndrome

G. AVANZINI, S. BINELLI, S. FRANCESCHETTI, F. PANZICA
and A. POZZI

*Department of Neurophysiology, 'C. Besta' National Neurological Institute,
Milan, Italy.*

INTRODUCTION

Bilateral and synchronous, but not necessarily symmetrical, myoclonic jerks on awakening are obligatory components of the clinical picture of Juvenile Myoclonic Epilepsy (JME), also called Janz syndrome, because it was first described by Dieter Janz in 1957 (Janz and Christian, 1957).

Human and animal studies have considerably advanced our understanding of the different pathophysiological mechanisms underlying the myoclonic phenomenology that occurs in various neurological diseases. Ultimately, the nerve cell discharge responsible for a jerk in a given group of muscles is located in their respective motoneurons. However, with the exception of spinal myoclonus, the activation of the motoneurons is secondary to a highly synchronized discharge that originates in other regions of the nervous system, and is subsequently transmitted to the motoneurons through the descending pathways. Thus, the olivo-dentato-rubro (or Mollaret's) triangle has been implicated in the pathophysiology of palatal myoclonus (Guillain and Mollaret, 1931), the caudal part of the medulla in the pathophysiology of reticular myoclonus (Hallet *et al.*, 1977), and the cerebral cortex (Hallet *et al.*, 1979), and basal ganglia in the myoclonic symptomatology associated with pathological situations (i.e. cortico-basal degeneration) affecting the neo-cortex and/or subcortical nuclei (Thompson *et al.*, 1994).

First carried out by Dawson (1946,1947), neurophysiological analysis of patients in whom myoclonus can be triggered by appropriate stimuli (reflex myoclonus) has identified the cerebral circuits potentially responsible for this special type of myoclonus. On the basis of the topography and latencies of muscle reflex jerks, and the time relationship between the jerks and their electroencephalographic (EEG) correlates, the myoclonus can be defined as a reticular (Hallet *et al.*, 1977) or cortical (Hallet *et al.*, 1979) reflex, although recent data suggest that other subcortical circuits may be involved in some cases that do not fit this definition (Cantello *et al.*, 1997). The general relevance of the criteria defining cortical, reticular or other subcortical types of reflex myoclonus to the pathophysiology of the apparently spontaneous awakening myoclonus that characterizes Janz syndrome has still to be evaluated.

As the techniques that have been developed to detect non-obvious EEG correlates of reflex myoclonus (e.g. the back-averaging procedure of Shibasaki and Kuroiwa, 1975) can be profitably be used to investigate Janz syndrome myoclonus, the first section of this chapter is devoted to the correlation between myoclonus and EEG discharges and will describe some of the results of such an investigation; the second section will concentrate on an attempt to analyse the relationship between EEG discharges and arousal-related EEG changes.

An association between spike-wave (SW)/polyspike-wave (PSW) complexes and arousal fluctuations of non-rapid eye movement (REM) sleep (cyclic alternating pattern: CAP, Terzano *et al.*, 1985) has been previously observed in JME patients by Gigli *et al.* (1992). The present authors' results will be interpreted with reference to the previous observations in order to evaluate the possible role of the neurophysiological mechanisms responsible for the unstable phases of the level of arousal in the pathophysiology of JME myoclonus.

SUBJECTS AND METHODS

Between 1993 and 1997, 33 patients with a definite diagnosis of JME underwent at least one computerized EEG recording at the Department of Neurophysiology of the Istituto Nazionale Neurologico 'C. Besta'; their main characteristics are summarized in Tables 1 and 2. The majority of patients were female (26/33); the ages at the time of the EEG examination ranged from 12 to 42 years. At the time of observation, all but eight of the patients were taking antiepileptic drug (AED) therapy. The occasional occurrence of awakening myoclonus was reported by all of the patients. Polygraphic recordings of myoclonus, invariably associated with bilateral EEG discharges of SW/PSW, were available for six patients, four of whom were not receiving antiepileptic therapy at the time of recording; the remaining two were on valproate and primidone respectively.

Twenty-eight patients had previously experienced at least one tonic-clonic seizure after awakening. The previous occurrence of childhood absence seizures was reported in the six cases marked (+) in Table 1; they were still

Table 1. Main clinical characteristics of the patients.

Patient no.	Age	Sex	Age at onset (years)	Awakening myoclonus	Tonic/ clonic seizures	Absences	Other	Therapy	Familial ante- cedents
1	16	F	10	+	+	–	–	VPA; PB	–
2	21	F	20	+	+	–	–	VPA	–
3	31	F	13	+	+	–	–	VPA; PB	–
4	37	F	13	+	–	–	–	VPA	+
5	15	F	15	+	–	–	–	–	–
6	27	M	16	+	+	–	–	VPA	–
7	42	F	13	+	+	–	–	PB	–
8	28	F	27	+	–	–	–	–	–
9	22	F	14	+	+	–	–	VPA	+
10	25	M	16	+	+	++	–	–	–
11	21	F	13	+	+	–	–	PB	–
12	34	F	12	+	+	–	FC 5 yrs	PB	+
13	20	F	12	+	+	(+)	–	VPA	–
14	29	M	16	+	+	–	–	VPA; PB	–
15	28	F	16	+	+	–	–	VPA	–
16	35	F	15	+	+	++	–	PHT; PB	–
17	15	F	15	+	+	–	–	–	+
18	15	F	15	+	+	(+)	–	–	–
19	37	F	20	+	+	–	–	VPA	+
20	18	F	14	+	+	–	–	CBZ	–
21	15	M	14	+	+	–	FC 5 mos	–	+
22	13	F	11	+	+	–	–	PRM	–
23	29	F	13	+	+	(+)	–	PB	–
24	16	M	15	+	+	(+)	–	VPA	–
25	24	F	12	+	+	++ (+)	–	VPA	+
26	13	F	13	+	+	–	FC (1 yr)	VPA	+
27	15	F	13	+	–	++	–	VPA	–
28	36	M	16	+	+	–	–	PB	–
29	16	F	16	+	–	(+)	–	VPA	–
30	12	F	15	+	+	–	–	–	–
31	17	M	12	+	+	–	–	–	+
32	30	F	16	+	+	–	–	PB	–
33	32	F	17	+	+	–	–	PB	–

(+), previous absence seizures; ++, absence seizures present at time of examination; FC, febrile convulsions; VPA, valproic acid; PB, phenobarbital; PHT, phenytoin; CBZ, carbamazepine; PRM, primidone.

present at the time of examination in a further four patients marked +. Febrile convulsions (FC) had occurred in three patients.

EEG analysis

EEG and electromyographic (EMG) recordings were retrieved from the archives of the Department of Neurophysiology, where they had been stored on optic disks.

Table 2. Main EEG data.

Patient no.	EEG		Interictal discharges	Ictal discharges	PPR
	Standard	Sleep			
1	–	+	–	–	–
2	+	–	+	–	–
3	+	–	+	–	–
4	+	–	–	–	–
5	+	–	+	+	+
6	–	+	+	–	+
7	+	–	–	–	–
8	–	+	+	–	–
9	+	–	–	–	–
10	+	+	+	–	–
11	+	–	–	–	–
12	–	+	+	–	–
13	+	–	–	–	–
14	+	+	+	–	–
15	–	+	+	–	–
16	+	–	–	–	–
17	–	+	+	–	+
18	–	+	+	+	+
19	+	–	–	–	–
20	–	+	+	–	–
21	–	+	+	+	–
22	–	+	+	+	+
23	+	–	+	–	–
24	–	+	+	–	–
25	+	–	+	–	+
26	+	–	–	–	–
27	+	–	+	–	+
28	–	+	+	–	+
29	–	+	+	+	–
30	–	+	+	+	+
31	+	–	+	–	–
32	–	+	+	–	–
33	–	+	–	–	–

–, not performed or not present; +, performed or present; PPR, photoparoxysmal response.

The EEG signals were recorded from Ag-AgCl scalp electrodes placed according to the International 10-20 System (band pass filter of 1.2–120 Hz); the EMG activity was simultaneously recorded from pairs of electrodes placed 2–3 cm apart over the belly of the left deltoid muscle.

The EEG and EMG signals were acquired and continuously stored on a Micromed computerized EEG system at a sampling frequency of 256 Hz. The EEGs were recorded using montages with a common reference electrode that allowed off-line mathematical data reformatting. The average common reference was used for jerk-locked averaging (JLA) analysis, whereas the evaluation of EEG and EMG signals was made on traces reformatted as conventional bipolar recordings. Nap recordings with a sleep depth never exceeding stage 3 of non REM sleep were available in 18 patients. The CAP sequences and their relationships to SW and PSW discharges were visually assessed using the polygraphic recording criteria of Terzano *et al.* (1985).

JLA procedure

Appropriate PC software detected and marked the occurrence of myoclonic triggering jerks on the rectified EMG signal, and displayed the EEG and EMG traces on the computer screen in such a way as to show an analysis window of 100 ms before the trigger point and 200 ms after it. Each epoch was visually reviewed in order to ensure the accurate identification of myoclonus onset and, at this time, it was possible to redefine manually the point at which the rectified EMG diverged from baseline (Barrett *et al.*, 1985). Only artefact-free single trials were selected for averaging.

Somatosensory evoked potentials

Upper-limb somatosensory evoked potentials were studied by means of electrical stimulation of the right and left median nerve at the wrist. A multi-channel recording was made from electrodes positioned on the Erb point, the seventh cervical spinous process, and on scalp centroparietal C_4' and C_3'. The stimulus frequency was 4.1 Hz.

RESULTS

Relationship between myoclonus and EEG discharges

In all but eight cases, the EEG recordings were obtained when the patients were receiving antiepileptic therapy. In the two patients (nos 21 and 22) for whom simultaneous recordings of the EEG discharges and myoclonus were available, the myoclonic jerks were invariably associated with SW and PSW. EEG discharges not associated with myoclonus (interictal) were recorded in 23 of the 33 cases. Both ictal and interictal EEG discharges consisted of bilateral arrhythmic SW and PSW, sometimes preceded by spiky 14–16 Hz activity of increasing amplitude (Figure 1(A)). The PSW amplitude was often asymmetrical (Figure 1(B)), with the extreme case being an occasional exclusively unilateral expression of PSW (Figure 1(C)). In 9 patients (five of whom were on antiepileptic therapy) SW–PSW were clearly evoked by intermittent light stimulation (Figure 1(D)). In order to better characterize the neurophysiology of myoclonus in Janz syndrome the JLA procedure (Shibasaki and Kuroiwa, 1975; Barrett *et al.*, 1985; Barrett 1992) was applied to the polygraphic signals recorded from the two patients (nos 21 and 22) in whom a sufficiently large

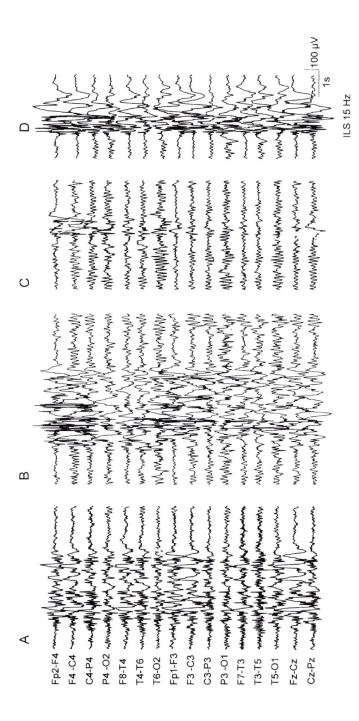

Figure 1. Representative examples of different patterns of interictal and ictal discharges in juvenile myoclonic epilepsy. (A) Bilateral and synchronous spike-wave/polyspike-wave (SW/PSW) discharge. Note the rhythmic 15 Hz activity of increasing amplitude preceding the onset of the discharge. (B) Bilateral synchronous SW/PSW with asymmetrical amplitude discharge more evident in the right anterior region. (C) Unilateral interictal SW discharge. (D) Photoparoxysmal response consisting of a bilateral SW/PSW discharge. ILS, intermittent light stimulation.

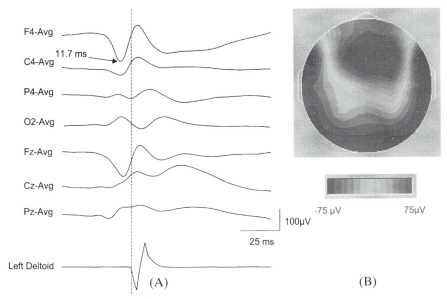

Figure 2. (A) Averaged EEG and EMG signals (26 epochs) in case no. 21. The EEG traces, time-locked to EMG onset, show a positive–negative sharp-wave in the right anterior regions that precedes the myoclonus onset in the left deltoid muscle by 11.7 ms. (B) Map of the initial peak of the cortical spike preceding myoclonus; the positive peak is maximal in the right and vertex frontocentral regions.

number of artefact-free EEG-EMG samples allowed a suitable analysis of the time relationship between myoclonic jerks and EEG discharges.

In both cases, JLA detected a positive–negative EEG sharp-wave in the frontocentral region contralateral to the myoclonus (Figures 2 and 3). The amplitude of the EEG transient was maximal in the frontal area, and the early positive peak of the cortical sharp-wave preceded the onset of EMG activity by respectively 11.7 and 15.6 ms.

In case no. 21, the anterior positive peak was clearly associated with a negative peak at the same latency in the parieto-occipital region, the maximal amplitude of which was on O_2; in case no. 22, it was associated with a negative shift of the potential in the posterior regions.

The somatosensory evoked potentials recorded in 2/8 cases not taking AEDs (nos 17 and 18) had a normal pattern.

Discharge expression and arousal-related EEG changes

A typical sequence of PSW discharges occurring 15 seconds after awakening and occasionally associated with myoclonias of the left deltoid in patient 24 is

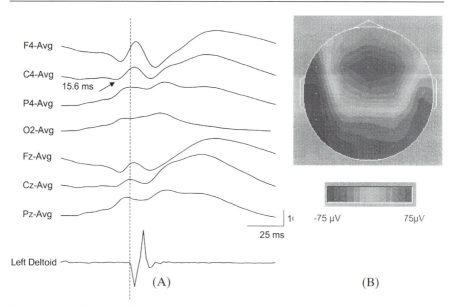

F4-Avg

C4-Avg
15.6 ms

P4-Avg

O2-Avg

Fz-Avg

Cz-Avg

Pz-Avg

1(-75 µV   75µV

25 ms

Left Deltoid

(A)   (B)

Figure 3. (A) Results of jerk-locked averaging in case no. 22. The positive peak of the spike in the central contralateral area precedes the onset of EMG activity by 15.6 ms. (B) Scalp topography map of the initial peak of the cortical spike preceding myoclonus; the positive peak is maximal in the right frontocentral region.

shown in Figure 4. In the EEG preceding the discharge a biphasic pattern with a large amplitude run (A) followed by a lower voltage, more homogeneous run (B) has been tentatively identified (Figure 5); the PSW discharges consistently coincided with the beginning of the former. The relationship between an awakening PSW discharge and phasic changes in EEG background activity was also present in the other patient (no. 22) from whom awakening PSWs were recorded.

In both patients, the correlation between the PSWs and the periodic fluctuations in the level of EEG activation revealed by CAPs (Terzano *et al.*, 1985) was evaluated during diurnal sleep episodes. The discharges were consistently found to be associated with A-type runs (Figure 6), very often in continuity with runs of spindles (Figure 7).

DISCUSSION

On the basis of their clinical features, all of the 33 patients considered here can be classified as having JME (Commission, 1989). In particular, they had all experienced awakening myoclonus that never occurred before the age of

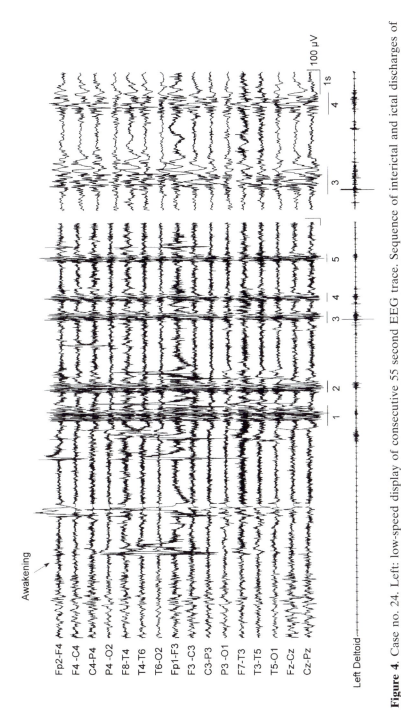

Figure 4. Case no. 24. Left: low-speed display of consecutive 55 second EEG trace. Sequence of interictal and ictal discharges of bilateral and synchronous spike-wave/polyspike-wave complexes occurring immediately after awakening. Right: higher-speed display of discharges 3 and 4.

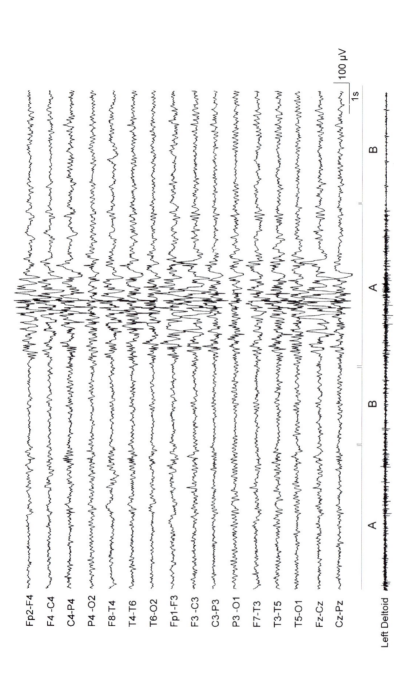

Figure 5. Case no. 24. Awakening polyspike-wave discharge. Two different EEG patterns marked A (larger EEG amplitude associated with greater EMG activity) and B (smaller EEG amplitude associated with less EMG activity) are tentatively identified.

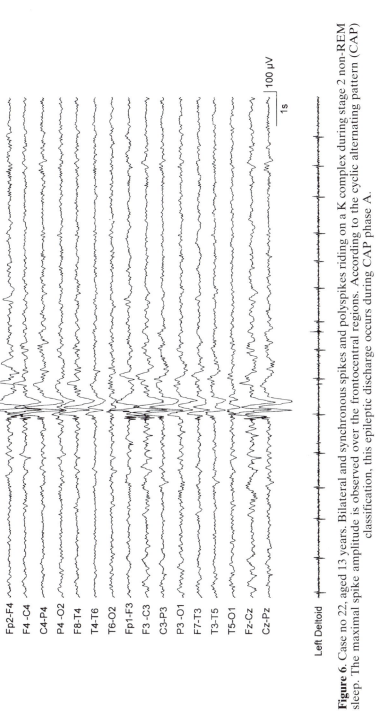

Figure 6. Case no 22, aged 13 years. Bilateral and synchronous spikes and polyspikes riding on a K complex during stage 2 non-REM sleep. The maximal spike amplitude is observed over the frontocentral regions. According to the cyclic alternating pattern (CAP) classification, this epileptic discharge occurs during CAP phase A.

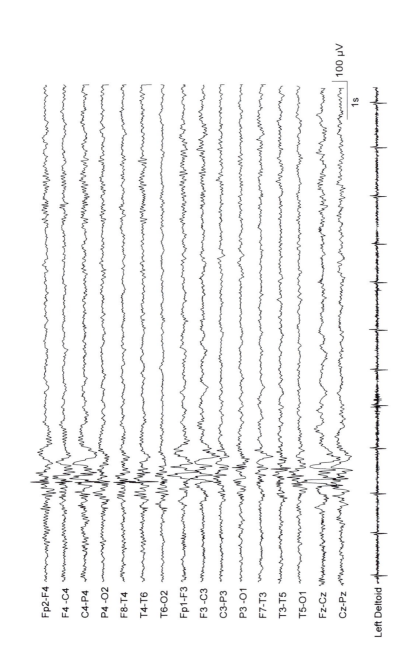

Figure 7. Case no. 24, aged 17 years. Spike and polyspikes superimposed on spindles and K complex, during stage 2, non-REM sleep.

10, with age at onset being between 11 and 15 years in 21 cases. In agreement with other data published in the literature (Delgado-Escueta and Enrile-Bacsal, 1984; Grünewald and Panayiotopoulos, 1993), familial antecedents were reported in more than one-third of the cases. All but four of the patients were seen in consultation because of the occurrence of tonic-clonic seizures (28 cases) or absences (one case). This corresponds to the general experience: most patients with JME tend to disregard the occasional awakening myoclonus and go to a physician only when some other type of seizure (usually tonic-clonic) occurs. Tonic-clonic seizures were reported by 28 patients, childhood absences by nine (in four aged from 12–16 years they were still present at the time of examination), and febrile convulsions by three. Photoparoxysmal responses were recorded from nine patients, a slightly lower proportion than that reported in the literature (Panayiotopoulos et al., 1994); this difference may have been due to the interference of AEDs. The higher percentage of females in this case series is considered to be casual.

Interictal SW/PSW discharges were recorded in 22 patients but ictal discharges (i.e. associated with myoclonus) could be recorded in only six, four of whom were not taking any AED.

The present analysis was therefore forcedly limited to six of the 33 cases. In the two cases studied by JLA, the latency of the EEG positive peak associated with the onset of left deltoid myoclonus was respectively 11.7 and 15.6 ms. The former was well within the time interval between the cortical magnetic stimulation and the activation of biceps and deltoids measured in normal subjects (Benecke et al., 1988; Dvorak et al, 1990; Rossini et al., 1994), whereas the latter was slightly longer than the usual upper limit.

The myoclonic jerks in these patients can therefore be attributed to the activation of the corticospinal system, although this does not rule out the possibility that the mechanisms underlying the cortical discharge which are ultimately responsible for the myoclonic jerks may involve subcortical (thalamic) structures. It has, in fact, long been recognized that generalized SW discharges are regulated by the thalamocortical system (Jasper and Droogleveer-Fortuyn, 1947) and that the corticosubcortical loop established by intrathalamic, thalamocortical (TC) and corticothalamic connections is consistently involved in their generation (Gloor and Fariello, 1988; de Curtis and Avanzini, 1994). Due to the intrinsic properties of thalamic nuclei, this circuit is particularly apt to sustain oscillatory activities relevant to physiological and pathological EEG rhythms. A crucial role is played by the low threshold T-type Ca^{2+} current first demonstrated in TC neurons by Jahnsen and Llinas (1984), and Steriade and Deschenes (1984), and further studied in reticular thalamic (Rt) neurons by Mulle et al. (1986), and Avanzini et al. (1989). The results obtained in the Genetic Absence Epilepsy Rat from Strasbourg (GAERS) by Avanzini et al. (1993) and Tsakiridou et al. (1995) suggest that a genetically determined overexpression of T-current in Rt neurons is responsible for the spontaneously occurring SW discharges in these animals. The contribution of the same circuitry in regulating the SW/PSW activities typically observed in JME should therefore be taken into account.

The TC oscillatory system involving Rt, TC relay nuclei and their mutual interconnection is known to be involved in the generation of the rhythmic activities associated with sleep (Steriade *et al.*, 1993). Therefore the analysis of the relationship between SW/PSW discharges and sleep rhythms may provide some insight into the specific contribution of thalamic structures to the discharge regulation. In agreement with those of a previous systematic study undertaken by Gigli *et al.* (1992), the present results show a consistent relationship between SW/PSW sequences and phase A of CAP segments that are considered to be the organism's response to protect sleep continuity from arousal stimuli (Terzano *et al.*, 1992; Gigli *et al.*, 1992). If this protective reaction involved activation of the oscillatory TC system, this would support the hypothesis of its involvement in SW-PSW regulation; furthermore, SW/PSW activity has been found in continuity with the sleep spindles that are known to be generated by the intrathalamic Rt-TC circuitry (Steriade *et al.*, 1993). One possible expression of SW/PSW-related activation of the TC oscillatory system is the finding of increasing 14–16 Hz activity heralding SW/PSW discharges.

In discussing their results Gigli *et al.* (1992) suggested that the marked facilitation of JME paroxysms after awakening might express a system instability that is comparable to that associated to CAP-related fluctuations in arousal. In the present authors' recordings, the occurrence of SW/PSW after awakening often correlated with phasic changes in background activity reminiscent of the two CAP phases A and B.

In conclusion, the authors' electrophysiological analysis demonstrates that the use of appropriate methods can lead to the detection of a highly synchronized time-locked cortical discharge which accounts for JME myoclonus. The present observations concur with previous results in supporting a role of a TC circuit in sustaining the repetitive discharge of SW/PSW typically observed in JME. It is suggested that arousal-related modulations of TC activities may facilitate the discharges typically observed in the transitional phases between sleep and awakening.

REFERENCES

Avanzini, G., de Curtis, M., Panzica, F. and Spreafico, R. (1989). Intrinsic properties of nucleus reticularis thalami neurones of the rat studied in vitro. *J Physiol* **416**, 111–122.

Avanzini, G., Vergnes, M., Spreafico, R. and Marescaux, C. (1993). Calcium-dependent regulation of genetically determined spike and wave by the reticular thalamic nucleus of rats. *Epilepsia* **34**, 1–7.

Barrett, G. (1992). Jerk-locked averaging: technique and application. *J Clin Neurophysiol* **9**, 495–508.

Barrett, G., Shibasaki, H. and Neshige, R. (1985). A computer-assisted method for averaging movement-related cortical potentials with respect to EMG onset. *Electroenceph Clin Neurophysiol* **60**, 276–281.

Benecke, R., Meyer, B.U., Gohmann, M. and Conrad, B. (1988). Analysis of muscle responses elicited by transcranial stimulation of the cortico-spinal system in man. *Electroenceph Clin Neurophysiol* **69**, 412–422.

Cantello, R., Giannelli, M., Civardi, C. and Mutani, R. (1997). Focal subcortical reflex myoclonus. *Arch Neurol* **54**, 187–196.

Commission on Classification and Terminology of the International League Against Epilepsy (1989). Proposal for revised classification of epilepsy and epileptic syndromes. *Epilepsia* **30**, 389–399.

Dawson, G.D. (1946). The relation between the electroencephalogram and muscle action potentials in certain convulsive states. *J Neurol Neurosurg Psychiatry* **9**, 5–22.

Dawson, G.D. (1947). Investigations on a patient subject to myoclonic seizures after sensory stimulation. *J Neurol Neurosurg Psychiatry* **10**, 141–162.

De Curtis, M. and Avanzini, G. (1994). Thalamic regulation of epileptic spike and wave discharges. *Funct Neurol* **9**, 307–326.

Delgado-Escueta, A.V. and Enrile-Bacsal, F.E. (1984). Juvenile myoclonic epilepsy of Janz. *Neurology* **34**, 285–294.

Dvorak, J., Herdmann, J. and Theiler, R. (1990). Magnetic transcranial brain stimulation: painless evaluation of central motor pathways; normal values and clinical application in spinal cord diagnostic: upper extremities. *Spine* **15**, 155–160.

Gigli, G.L., Calia, E., Marciani, M.G. *et al.* (1992). Sleep microstructure and EEG epileptiform activity in patients with juvenile myoclonic epilepsy. *Epilepsia* **33**, 799–804.

Gloor, P. and Fariello, R.G. (1988). Generalized epilepsy: some of its cellular mechanisms differ from those of focal epilepsy. *Trends Neurosci* **11**, 63–68.

Grünewald, R.A. and Panayiotopoulos, C.P. (1993). Juvenile myoclonic epilepsy. A review. *Arch Neurol* **50**, 594–598.

Guillain, G. and Mollaret, P. (1931). Deux cas de myoclonies synchrones et rythmées vélo-pharyngo-laryngo-oculo-diaphragmatiques. Le problème anatomique et physio-pathologique de ce syndrom. *Rev Neurol* **2**, 545–566.

Hallet, M., Chadwick, D., Adam, J. and Marsden, C.D. (1977). Reticular reflex myoclonus. *J Neurol Neurosurg Psychiatry* **40**, 253–264.

Hallet, M., Chadwick, D. and Marsden, C.D. (1979). Cortical reflex myoclonus. *Neurology* **29**, 1107–1125.

Jahnsen, H. and Llinas, R. (1984). Ionic basis for the electroresponsiveness and oscillatory properties of guinea-pig thalamic neurones in vitro. *J Physiol* **349**, 227–247

Janz, D. Christian, W. (1957). Impulsive-petit mal. *Dtsch Z. Nervenheilk* **176**, 346–386.

Jasper, H.H. and Droogleveer-Fortuyn, J., (1947). Experimental studies of the functional anatomy of the petit mal epilepsy. *Assoc Res Nerv Ment Disord Proc* **26**, 272–298.

Mulle, C., Madariaga, A. and Deschenes, M., (1986). Morphology and electrophysiological properties of RT neurons in the cat: in vivo study of a thalamic pacemaker. *J Neurosci* **6**, 2134–2145.

Panayiotopoulos, C.P., Obeid, T. and Tahan, A.R. (1994). Juvenile myoclonic epilepsy: a 5-year prospective study. *Epilepsia* **35**, 285–296.

Rossini, P.M., Barker, A.T., Berardelli, A. *et al.* (1994). Non-invasive electrical and magnetic stimulation of the brain, spinal cord and roots: basic principles and procedures for routine clinical application. Report of an IFCN Committee. *Electroenceph Clin Neurophysiol* **91**: 79–92.

Shibasaki, H. and Kuroiwa, Y. (1975). Electroencephalographic correlates of myoclonus. *Electroenceph Clin Neurophysiol* **39**, 455–463.

Steriade, M. and Deschenes, M. (1984). The thalamus as a neuronal oscillator. *Brain Res Rev* **8**, 1–63.

Steriade, M., McCormick, D.A. and Sejnowski, T.J. (1993). Thalomocortical oscillations in the sleeping and aroused brain. *Science* **262**, 679–685.

Terzano, M.G., Mancia, D., Salati, M.R., Costani, G., Decembrino, A. and Parrino, L. (1985). The cyclic alternating pattern as a physiologic component of normal NREM sleep. *Sleep* **8**, 137–145.

Terzano, M.G., Parrino, L., Floriti, G., Spaggiari, M.C. and Piroli, A. (1986). Morphologic and functional features of cyclic alternating pattern (CAP) sequences in normal REM sleep. *Funct Neurol* **1**, 29–41.

Terzano, M.G., Parrino, L., Anelli, S., Boselli, M. and Clemens, B. (1992). Effects of generalized interictal EEG discharges on sleep stability: assessment by means of cyclic alternating pattern. *Epilepsia* **33**, 317–326.

Thompson, P.D., Day, B.L., Rothwell, J.C., Brown, P., Britton, T.C. and Marsden, C.D. (1994). The myoclonus in corticobasal degeneration. Evidence for two forms of cortical reflex myoclonus. *Brain* **117**, 1197–1207.

Tsakiridou, E., Bertollini, L., de Curtis, M., Avanzini, G. and Pape, H.-C. (1995). Selective increase in T-type calcium conductance of reticular thalamic neurons in a rat model of absence epilepsy. *J Neurosci* **15**, 3110–3117.

Juvenile Myoclonic Epilepsy: The Janz Syndrome
Edited by Bettina Schmitz and Thomas Sander
© 2000 Wrightson Biomedical Publishing Ltd

7

Juvenile Myoclonic Epilepsy with Praxis-Induced Seizures

YUSHI INOUE and HIDEMOTO KUBOTA

National Epilepsy Centre, Shizuoka Higashi Hospital, Shizuoka, Japan

INTRODUCTION

Almost all patients with juvenile myoclonic epilepsy (JME) have seizure-precipitating factors. The well known factors (general factors) are sleep deprivation, irregular lifestyle or simple finger manipulation, and the seizures predominantly occur on awakening, as described by Janz and Christian (1957). Typically, JME patients have seizures when they engage in manual movements such as brushing their teeth, using a fork or chopsticks, or when changing or buttoning their clothes in the morning hours after lack of sleep. Moreover, there are patients whose seizures are easily induced by exposure to bright light or patterns, or their frequent changes, in addition to the general factors described above.

However, some JME patients may have another type of precipitation. They are sensitive to situations where they are obliged to contemplate complicated spatial tasks in a sequential fashion, to make decisions, and to respond practically by using a part of their body under stressful circumstances. The authors conceptualized such situations as praxis activity (Inoue *et al.*, 1994). These precipitating factors include ideation or execution of complicated movements involving sequential spatial processing such as calculation, playing games, drawing, writing, construction and complicated finger manipulation.

The authors divided the JME patients according to their precipitation and compared clinical and laboratory results in each in order to reveal possible differences existing between them.

SUBJECTS AND METHODS

The subjects were 213 JME patients whom the authors had treated over the previous seven years. Mean age at examination was 25.8 years (range 7–61), and the age at seizure onset was 13.4 years (range 4–29). There were 112 males and 101 females. Thirty-nine patients (18.3%) had a family history of epilepsy and 45 patients (21%) had family members who suffered occasional seizures, including febrile convulsions, in up to four-degree relatives. Sixty patients (28.2%) experienced febrile convulsions. Five patients had head trauma, seven had asphyxia, and one had meningitis before the onset of epilepsy.

As regards seizure precipitation, 130 patients, or 61%, had sleep deprivation or simple handling as seizure-precipitating factors (general factors). Twenty-three patients experienced environmental photosensitivity, and 27 patients had praxis sensitivity. Thirty-eight patients had occasional or incidental seizures precipitated by praxis activity, of whom five were also photosensitive.

The authors examined photosensitivity with an electroencephalogram (EEG) using a Grass PS33 photostimulator (Astro-Med, RI, USA) at a distance of 30 cm, with an intensity of 8 and frequencies ranging from 6 to 33 Hz. The patients were examined with eyes open, eye closure, and eyes closed. Pattern sensitivity was also examined, with black and white gratings shown for 10 seconds. Photosensitivity refers to photoparoxysmal responses (PPR), to intermittent photic stimulation (IPS), or patterns, defined as type 3 or type 4 by Waltz et al. (1992). Type 3 PPR is defined as parieto-occipital spikes with a biphasic slow wave and a spread to the frontal region, and type 4 as generalized spike/polyspike(s) and waves. Twenty-four patients showed EEG photosensitivity, without experiencing subjective photosensitivity in daily life. Ten patients showed both EEG and environmental photosensitivity. Of these 34 patients, 28 had type 4 PPR and the discharge continued after the disappearance of IPS in 26 patients. Together with 13 patients who had environmental photosensitivity but not EEG photosensitivity, 47 patients were recognized as photosensitive subjects.

The JME patients were therefore classified, according to their specific precipitation, into three groups: no precipitation (none) group ($n=110$), photosensitive group ($n=47$), and praxis-sensitive group ($n=27$). The remaining 29 patients with occasional or incidental praxis sensitivity and without environmental or EEG photosensitivity were excluded from the analysis. As indicated before, the 'none' group had general factors as precipitation. No patient in the praxis-sensitive group showed EEG photosensitivity. The authors examined the demographic and symptomatological features of the three groups and the responses to medical treatment of patients receiving antiepileptic drugs, and followed their condition for more than three years (134 patients).

Magnetoencephalography (MEG) was performed on 12 patients. Dual sensors were used, each of which consisted of a 37-channel gradiometer (Magnes & Magnes II, BTi, San Diego). Equivalent current dipoles (ECD) were estimated in order to localize the brain signal sources (Watanabe *et al.*, 1996). The sensory evoked potentials (SEP) in 65 patients were then examined according to the conventional method, with a total of 128 averaging and 200 ms analysis time. Monophasic square wave stimulation of 1 Hz and 0.2 ms duration was applied to the unilateral median nerve with an intensity 10% above the movement threshold. An EEG was recorded on the bilateral Shagass points with ear electrode as a reference, using a 3 kHz high cut and a 0.5 Hz low cut. The SEP waveform was analysed with amplitude (P24-N33) and latency from N20 to N60. Twenty healthy subjects served as a control.

Statistical analysis was performed using the chi-square method.

RESULTS

Praxis precipitation

The most common precipitation was writing or typing (20 patients), followed by playing cards or chess (16 patients), calculation or performing mathematics (15 patients), construction or drawing (11 patients), complicated finger manipulation (11 patients), playing video-games (six patients), and playing musical instruments (four patients). Stress and concentration were important accompanying factors. In two patients, reading or speaking also induced a seizure.

Demographic features (Table 1)

The onset age was the same for the three groups. There were more males in the praxis-sensitive group than in the other groups. Epilepsy in the family was slightly more common in the photosensitive group, but a history of occasional seizures was slightly more common in the praxis-sensitive group (nonsignificant).

Table 1. Demographic features.

Precipitation	n	Onset age (years)	Male : female	Epilepsy in the family	History of febrile convulsions
None (general factors)	110	13.1	57 : 53	17 (15.5%)	29 (26.4%)
Photosensitive	47	14.0	24 : 23	14 (29.8%)	10 (21.3%)
Praxis sensitive	27	13.4	19 : 8	6 (22.2%)	11 (40.7%)

Table 2. Precipitation and seizure types.

Precipitation	n	Myoclonias	Absences	GTCS
None (general factors)	110	110	15 (13.6%)	97 (88.2%)
Photosensitive	47	47	7 (14.9%)	42 (89.4%)
Praxis sensitive	27	27	9 (33.3%)	26 (96.3%)

GTCS, generalized tonic-clonic seizures.

Seizure types (Table 2)

As per the definition, all patients had myoclonias. Absence seizures were more often observed in the praxis-sensitive group than in the no-precipitation group ($p < 0.05$) and generalized tonic-clonic seizures (GTCS) occurred slightly more often in the praxis-sensitive group.

Treatment results (Table 3)

A seizure-free interval of less than three years was slightly more common in patients in the praxis-sensitive group, and photosensitive patients generated slightly less favourable results than the no-precipitation group. Valproate (102 patients) or clonazepam (71 patients), or both, were the drugs most often taken, followed by phenobarbital (19 patients), phenytoin (19 patients), zonisamide (four patients), and acetazolamide (two patients), often in combination with either valproate or clonazepam.

Table 3. Treatment results.

Precipitation	n	Seizure-free interval	
		>3 years	<3 years
None (general factors)	77	53 (69%)	24 (31%)
Photosensitive	32	18 (56%)	14 (44%)
Praxis sensitive	25	12 (48%)	13 (52%)

MEG study (Table 4)

In patients with photosensitivity or praxis sensitivity, MEG spike dipoles tended to localize in a certain area or lobe. In general, the spike dipoles of photosensitive patients were distributed more over the posterior, and those of the praxis-sensitive patients more over the anterior part of the brain.

Table 4. Magnetoencephalography.

Precipitation	n	Dipole localization of interictal spikes
None (general factors)	2	Bilateral frontal, widely distributed
		Bilateral frontal, widely distributed
Photosensitive	6	Right frontal
		Right frontal
		Right frontoparietal
		Left frontoparietal
		Bilateral parieto-occipital
		Bilateral parieto-occipital, right frontal
Praxis sensitive	4	Left frontal
		Left frontal
		Left frontal
		Right frontoparietal

SEP study (Table 5)

There was no difference in latency between the normal control and JME patients. However, amplitude (P24 minus N33) was significantly higher in JME patients than in the controls. JME patients with photosensitivity or praxis sensitivity had a significantly higher amplitude than those without.

Table 5. Sensory evoked potentials of juvenile myoclonic epilepsy (JME) patients compared with healthy subjects.

	n	Age (years)	P24–N33 (SD) (μV)	p vs control	p vs NP
Control	20	34.6	2.82 (1.43)	–	–
JME	65	25.6	4.07 (2.16)	<0.05	–
No precipitation (NP)	25	28.4	3.38 (1.78)	0.26	–
Photosensitive	20	22.5	4.65 (2.35)	<0.01	<0.05
Praxis sensitive	11	25.6	4.92 (2.48)	<0.01	<0.05

SD, standard deviation.

ILLUSTRATIVE CASES

Case 1

A 16-year-old left-handed male with a febrile convulsion at age two. He had a distant relative with epilepsy. Weekly myoclonic seizures started at age 14 and he experienced five GTCS preceded by repetitive myoclonias. He had an IQ of 74 and the result of the Wisconsin card-sorting test (WCST) was poor (achieved category 0). His seizures occurred predominantly when he was captivated by playing chess, video games, or performing computer graphics. The EEG shows bursts of irregular fast spike- or polyspike-waves and

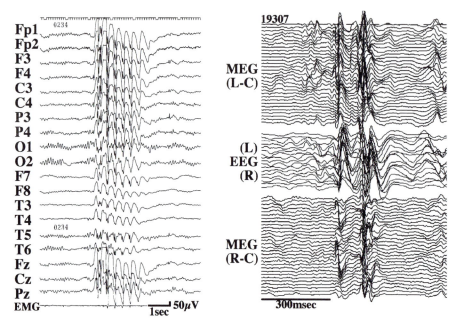

Figure 1. Interictal EEG (left) and MEG (right) of Case 1.

the left side MEG spikes always precede those of the right (Figure 1). His EEG was not sensitive to IPS. MEG spike dipoles clustered on the left frontal area. The SEP amplitude of P24–N33 was 8.75 with normal latency. He is receiving clonazepam, in addition to valproate, and has occasional seizures especially when noncompliant with medication.

Case 2

A 14-year-old student. He had three febrile convulsions at the age of one. At age 13, myoclonic seizures began. Myoclonia occurred predominantly in the right hand, resulting in the patient throwing away whatever he was holding. Sometimes the knee was involved, and he fell down. Myoclonia occurred twice a week, often precipitated by activities such as writing, calculating or playing video games. Myoclonias of the upper extremities evolved to generalized convulsions on four occasions.

Neuropsychological testing revealed an average IQ of 87, but the WCST result was poor (achieved category 2), and the results of verbal fluency and trail-making tests were below average, suggesting a dysfunction of the frontal lobe.

The EEG showed irregular spike-waves, with the highest amplitude on the left side and over the central area, but sometimes on the right side (Figure

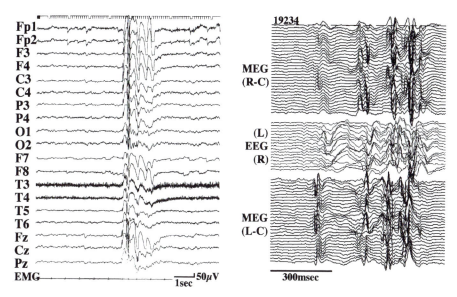

Figure 2. Interictal EEG (left) and MEG (right) of Case 2.

2, left). The EEG discharges appeared most often during writing, followed by written calculation, mental calculation, and video games. The SEP amplitude of P24–N33 was 6.56 with normal latency.

The MEG findings were constant in that the MEG spikes of the left hemisphere preceded those of the right (Figure 2, right). Ictal MEG also showed that the spikes appeared on the left side first. The MEG spike dipole cluster was predominantly in the left frontal region interictally, as well as ictally. SPECT indicated a lowered perfusion on the left anterior region, although MRI was normal.

He has been seizure-free for more than three years using valproate.

DISCUSSION

Photosensitivity and praxis sensitivity are distinct precipitations in patients with JME. The patients are aware of the seizure induction by these factors and often try to avoid them. The feasibility of seizure induction can be shown with EEGs activated by IPS or by neuropsychological tasks. The SEP examination showed higher amplitudes in patients with photosensitivity or praxis sensitivity than those without. This fact suggests that photosensitivity and praxis sensitivity may reflect an increased excitability of the cortex in JME patients.

There were minimal differences in the clinical and demographic features between the photosensitive and the praxis-sensitive patients. The praxis-sensitive patients had a slightly higher ratio of males and more frequent absence seizures, and treatment results were slightly less favourable. Most of these differences did not reach a statistically significant level, and other features such as the onset age were almost identical.

However, photosensitivity and praxis sensitivity seem to stand in clear contrast. Patients with praxis sensitivity as the main precipitation did not show EEG photosensitivity, and only nine photosensitive patients (environmental, three; EEG, four; both environmental and EEG, two) showed occasional or incidental praxis sensitivity in our sample. This distinction was supported by the results of the MEG study. In patients with praxis-sensitivity, MEG spike dipoles tended to distribute more over the anterior part of the brain (mainly premotor or posterior prefrontal areas) than in photosensitive patients. The involvement of the anterior part of the cortex in praxis-sensitive patients is suggested by the neuropsychological test results and single photon emission computerized tomography findings in cases 1 and 2, although these findings were anecdotal because a systematic study was not carried out. Despite the small sample size, these results suggest that photosensitivity and praxis sensitivity may represent a spatially different excitability of the cortex.

JME is not the only epilepsy with praxis sensitivity or photosensitivity. These precipitations probably reflect regional brain dysfunctions which are vulnerable to epileptic bombardment. The authors conclude that JME may have focal or regionally accentuated cortical vulnerability that eventually activates a generalized epileptogenic mechanism. In praxis sensitivity, the most affected region may be in either the frontal lobe or the parietal lobe, as suggested by Goossens et al. (1990).

CONCLUSION

Praxis sensitivity represents an important precipitating factor in patients with JME. Of 213 JME patients, 27 were praxis-sensitive. These patients were often male, having infrequent photosensitivity. Absence seizures were observed more often than in other JME patients. They were inclined to resist medical therapy. MEG spike dipoles tended to distribute more over the anterior part of the brain than in photosensitive patients. SEP amplitude was higher than in controls and JME patients without specific precipitation. These results suggest that praxis sensitivity may represent a more excitable, and probably focally accentuated pathology of JME, similar to photosensitivity. The distinction between praxis sensitivity and photosensitivity may reflect a difference in spatial distribution of the excitable cortex.

REFERENCES

Goossens, L., Andermann, F., Andermann, E. and Remillard, G.M. (1990). Reflex seizures induced by calculation, card or board games, and spatial tasks: a review of 25 patients and delineation of the epileptic syndromes. *Neurology* **40**, 1171–1176.

Inoue, Y., Seino, M., Kubota, H., Yamakaku, K., Tanaka, M. and Yagi, K. (1994). Epilepsy with praxis-induced seizures. In: Wolf, P. (Ed.), *Epileptic Seizures and Syndromes*, John Libbey, London. pp. 81–91.

Janz, D. and Christian, W. (1957). Impulsive petit mal. *J Neurol* **176**, 346–386.

Waltz, S., Christen, H.J. and Doose, H. (1992). The different patterns of the photoparoxysmal response: a genetic study. *Electroencephalogr Clin Neurophysiol* **83**, 138–145.

Watanabe, Y., Fukao, K., Watanabe, M. and Seino, M. (1996). Epileptic events observed by multichannel MEG. In: Hashimoto, I., Okada, Y.C. and Ogawa, S. (Eds), *Visualization of Information Processing in the Human Brain: Recent Advances in MEG and Functional MRI* (EEG Suppl. 47), Elsevier, Oxford, pp. 383–392.

8

Structural Changes in Juvenile Myoclonic Epilepsy: Evidence from Quantitative MRI

FRIEDRICH G. WOERMANN and JOHN S. DUNCAN

University Department of Clinical Neurology, Institute of Neurology, London, UK

INTRODUCTION

Juvenile myoclonic epilepsy (JME) is a syndrome of idiopathic generalized epilepsy with an age-related onset of seizures; it is characterized by myoclonic jerks, tonic-clonic seizures and, less frequently, by typical absences. Prevalence is 5–10% amongst adult and adolescent patients with epilepsies, and both sexes are equally affected (Janz and Durner, 1997). As with other syndromes of idiopathic generalized epilepsy, JME is defined by electrophysiological features indicating involvement of both cerebral hemispheres from the beginning of seizures. Nevertheless, the 1989 definition of age-related idiopathic generalized epilepsies states that 'The patient usually has a normal interictal state, without neurologic or neuroradiologic signs' (Commission on Classification and Terminology of the ILAE, 1989).

In fact, routine magnetic resonance imaging (MRI) is normal on visual assessment in almost all patients with idiopathic generalized epilepsy and in patients with JME. With pathological studies of JME being very rare, there is no macroscopic correlate on imaging or pathology to the minimal malformations of cortical development described by Janz and Meencke (Janz and Neimanis, 1961; Meencke and Janz, 1984; Meencke, 1985) and discussed controversially by Lyon and Gastaut (1985). The recent finding that patients with periventricular nodular heterotopias visible on MRI can present with seizure disorders resembling idiopathic generalized epilepsy (Raymond *et al.*, 1994; Dubeau *et al.*, 1995; Fish, 1995) raised the possibility that more common phenotypes of idiopathic generalized epilepsy may be associated with subtle malformations of cortical development. As a rarity in idiopathic generalized epilepsy, these infrequent macroscopic abnormalities may, however, be chance findings just like the other macroscopic structural brain abnormalities in patients apparently suffering from primarily generalized seizures, described in the literature (see, for example, Stewart and Dreifuss, 1967; Stevens, 1970).

It was necessary to conduct quantitative imaging studies in groups of otherwise normal patients with idiopathic generalized epilepsy and JME to demonstrate the possibility that these patients may have structural cranial and cerebral abnormalities.

PREVIOUS KNOWLEDGE FROM SKULL X-RAYS AND OUTER BRAIN CONTOURS

An early study of quantitation used skull X-rays and compared a clinically well defined group of 33 patients with JME (*'Aufwachepilepsie mit Impulsiv-Petit mal'*) with patients suffering from other epileptic syndromes (*n* = 135) and normal controls (*n* = 100) (Kammerer, 1961). Thus, not only comparing measures with control data, but in an attempt to control for nonspecific sequelae of epilepsy and antiepileptic treatment, Kammerer found that the frontal skull was thicker in patients with JME. These descriptive measures were meant to add to the classification of the epilepsies which at the time tried to integrate clinical, biological and constitutional data (Janz and Christian, 1957; Helmchen, 1958). Methodological problems of this study included patient selection, projectional errors in X-ray imaging and quantitation, and the fact that the finding of increased skull thickness was not described statistically; in addition, the use of multiple comparisons of numerous, nonindependent measures were not taken into account. The aetiological meaning of these findings remains unclear.

Moving in from the skull, a recent study of Savic *et al.* (1998) described distortions of the outer brain contours in patients suffering from generalized seizures. Using an interactive atlas-based fitting of outer brain contours derived from single planes in computerized tomography (CT) or MRI data, both male and female patients who suffered from generalized tonic-clonic seizures were compared with a group of male control subjects. The contour distortions were explained by an elongation or increase of volume in the frontal lobes and/or an atrophy of the cerebellum. This study used data from imaging modalities with different graphical distortions for rater-driven comparisons, and investigated selected patients, none of whom was diagnosed as suffering from a specific subsyndrome of idiopathic generalized epilepsy, such as JME.

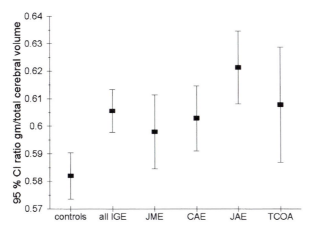

Figure 1. Mean normalized grey matter volumes (black squares) in the control group, all patients with idiopathic generalized epilepsy (IGE), and the subsyndromes. The bars indicate the 95% confidence interval. JME, juvenile myoclonic epilepsy; CAE, childhood absence epilepsy; JAE, juvenile absence epilepsy; TCOA, tonic-clonic seizures on awakening. (Reproduced with permission, from Woermann *et al.*, 1998a.)

QUANTITATIVE CEREBRAL MRI STUDIES IN IDIOPATHIC GENERALIZED AND JUVENILE MYOCLONIC EPILEPSY

In a recent study, 45 patients with idiopathic generalized epilepsy, including 20 patients with JME and 30 age- and sex-matched control subjects were scanned using a 1.5 T GE Signa MRI scanner (General Electrics, Milwaukee, USA) (Woermann *et al.*, 1998a). Using an interactive anatomical segmentation technique and volume of interest measurements in quantitative MRI, patients with idiopathic generalized epilepsy were shown to have significantly larger cortical grey matter volumes than control subjects (Figure 1). The normalized white matter volume was significantly lower compared with control subjects. Further, 40% of individual patients with JME had significant abnormalities of cerebral structure.

In this study (Woermann *et al.*, 1998a) a quantitative MRI method was applied to patients with idiopathic generalized epilepsy building on previous work from this group validating this approach. Before being used in patients with idiopathic generalized epilepsy, the same method of MRI quantitation demonstrated widespread structural cerebral changes not visible on high-resolution MRI in patients with apparently focal cerebral dysgenesis – with the identification of abnormalities beyond the visualized lesions (Sisodiya *et al.*, 1995). Similar widespread extratemporal structural changes were also correlated with an unfavourable outcome after anterior temporal lobe resections in patients with temporal lobe epilepsy and hippocampal sclerosis, thus connect-

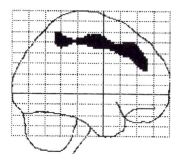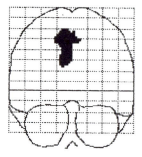

Figure 2. The sagittal and coronal glass brain views show those voxels with a significant increase of grey matter in the group of 20 patients with juvenile myoclonic epilepsy compared with 30 controls (thresholded for display, $p < 0.05$). (Reproduced with permission, from Woermann *et al.*, 1998b.)

ing these volumetric findings with epileptogenicity (Sisodiya and Free, 1997). Sisodiya *et al.* (1995) have previously postulated that these structural changes detected on MRI quantitation are possibly due to changes in neuronal connectivity. The basic tenet is that neocortical grey matter volumes allow inferences to be drawn about the number of cellular elements in these structures, especially those contributing to the neuropil (Caviness *et al.*, 1996). It is not known, however, whether similar quantitative MRI abnormalities in patients with partial seizures and malformations of cortical development and in patients with idiopathic generalized epilepsy are due to the same specific anatomical structural changes. Pathological studies are needed to address this question.

The spatial resolution of the above study (Woermann *et al.*, 1998a) was constrained by the use of predetermined volumes of interest. In a recent study, the new method was used of voxel-based morphometry and the automated and objective technique of statistical parametric mapping was applied to the analysis of structural MRI from 20 patients with JME and 30 normal subjects (Woermann *et al.*, 1998b). The cortical grey matter of each individual patient and control subject were normalized to Talairach space and smoothed before being compared on a voxel-by-voxel basis; this method had been validated for structural, semi-automatically segmented MRI in patients with macroscopic malformations of cortical development (Richardson *et al.*, 1997). Each individual patient and the group of patients were compared with the group of 30 normal subjects and the results were correlated with the findings of the previous volume of interest technique. The group comparison between patients and control subjects showed an increase of cortical grey matter in the mesial frontal lobes in JME (Figure 2). Analysis of individual patients revealed significant abnormalities of cortical grey matter in five out of 20 patients with JME, four of whom had widespread abnormalities using the previous volume of interest-based technique.

In the light of previous pathological, EEG, psychological and functional imaging findings, the demonstration of structural cerebral abnormalities in patients with JME using quantitative MRI might indicate an involvement of mesiofrontal cortical structures in the pathophysiology of the condition. The authors' findings of abnormal voxel-based MRI quantitation in JME are a possible structural correlate of the functional abnormalities in patients with idiopathic generalized epilepsy and JME shown recently. EEG studies have suggested that generalized epileptiform activity in idiopathic generalized epilepsy is generated in the (mesio-) frontal cortex (Rodin and Ancheta, 1987; Niedermeyer, 1996). Although some depth EEG studies in humans with idiopathic generalized epilepsy found discharges starting in the thalamus before the neocortex (Williams, 1953; Velasco et al., 1989), other studies failed to provide evidence of a primary thalamic onset in patients with generalized spike-wave complexes (Niedermeyer et al., 1969). Integrating animal data and clinical studies in patients with idiopathic generalized epilepsy supports the view that cortical hyperexcitability has an important part in the pathophysiology of idiopathic generalized epilepsy (Gloor, 1995). Patients with JME had a deficit in performance on a task of working memory that was nearly as severe as that of a group with frontal lobe epilepsy with or without obvious structural frontal lobe lesions (Swartz et al., 1994). A positron-emission tomography (PET) study investigating the same paradigm showed an association between impaired visual working memory and reduced 18-F-fluorodeoxyglucose uptake in various frontal cortical areas of patients with JME (Swartz et al., 1996). In a recent 11-C-flumazenil PET study, globally increased benzodiazepine receptor density was found in cerebral neocortex, thalamus and cerebellum of patients with JME that was consistent with increased neuronal density (Koepp et al., 1997).

CONCLUSION

Studies using MRI quantitation in patients with JME support the concept that structural cortical changes may be associated with abnormalities in functional connectivity within the mesiofrontal neocortex and between cortical and subcortical structures.

REFERENCES

Caviness, V.S., Kennedy, D.N., Bates, J.F. and Makris, N. (1996). The developing human brain: a morphometric profile. In: Thatcher, R.W., Reid Lyon, G., Rumsey, J. and Krasnegor, N. (Eds), *Developmental Neuroimaging. Mapping the Development of Brain and Behavior*, Academic Press, San Diego, CA, pp. 3–14.

Commission on Classification and Terminology of the ILAE (1989). Proposal for revised classification of epilepsies and epileptic syndromes. *Epilepsia* **30**, 389–399.

Dubeau, F., Tampieri, D., Lee, N. *et al.* (1995). Periventricular and subcortical nodular heterotopia. A study of 33 patients. *Brain* **118**, 1273–1287.

Fish, D.R. (1995). Blank spells that are not typical absences. In: Duncan, J.S. and Panayiotopoulous, C.P., (Eds), *Typical Absences and Related Epileptic Syndromes.* Churchill Communications Europe, London, pp. 253–259.

Gloor, P. (1995). Feline generalised penicillin epilepsy: extrapolations to neurophysiological mechanisms in humans. In: Duncan, J.S. and Panayiotopoulos, C.P. (Eds), *Typical Absences and Related Epileptic Syndromes.* Churchill Communications Europe, London, pp. 74–82.

Helmchen, H. (1958). Beitrag zur konstitutionellen Differenzierung im Bereich genuiner Epilepsien. *J Neurol* **179**, 541–582.

Janz, D. and Christian, W. (1957). Impulsiv-Petit mal. *J Neurol* **176**, 346–386.

Janz, D. and Durner, M. (1997). Juvenile myoclonic epilepsy. In: Engel, J. and Pedley, T.A. (Eds), *Epilepsy: A Comprehensive Textbook.* Lippincott-Raven, Philadelphia, pp. 2389–2400.

Janz, D. and Neimanis, G. (1961). Clinico-anatomical study of a case of idiopathic epilepsy with impulsive petit mal and grand mal on awakening. *Epilepsia* **2**, 251–269.

Kammerer, T. (1961). Untersuchungen am Schädelröntgenbild bei genuiner Epilepsie. *J Neurol* **182**, 13–33.

Koepp, M.J., Richardson, M.P., Brooks, D.J., Cunningham, V.J. and Duncan, J.S. (1997). Central benzodiazepine/GABAa receptors in idiopathic generalised epilepsy: an 11C-flumazenil PET study. *Epilepsia* **38**, 1089–1097.

Lyon, G. and Gastaut, H. (1985). Considerations on the significance attributed to unusual cerebral histological findings recently described in eight patients with primary generalized epilepsy. *Epilepsia* **26**, 365–367.

Meencke, H.J. (1985). Neuron density in the molecular layer of the frontal cortex in primary generalized epilepsy. *Epilepsia* **26**, 450–454.

Meencke, H.J. and Janz, D. (1984). Neuropathological findings in primary generalized epilepsy: a study of eight cases. *Epilepsia* **25**, 8–21.

Niedermeyer, E. (1996). Primary (idiopathic) generalized epilepsy and underlying mechanisms. *Clin Electroencephalogr* **27**, 1–21.

Niedermeyer, E., Laws, E.R. and Walker, A.E. (1969). Depth EEG findings in epileptics with generalized spike-wave complexes. *Arch Neurol* **21**, 51–58.

Raymond, A.A., Fish, D.R., Stevens, J.M., Sisodiya, S.M., Alsanjari, N. and Shorvon, S.D. (1994). Subependymal heterotopia: a distinct neuronal migration disorder associated with epilepsy. *J Neurol Neurosurg Psychiatry* **57**, 1195–1202.

Richardson, M.P., Friston, K.J., Sisodiya, S.M. *et al.* (1997). Cortical grey matter and benzodiazepine receptors in malformations of cortical development – a voxel-based comparison of structural and functional imaging data. *Brain* **120**, 1961–1973.

Rodin, E. and Ancheta, O. (1987). Cerebral electrical fields during petit mal absences. *Electroencephalogr Clin Neurophysiol* **66**, 457–466.

Savic, I., Seitz, R.J. and Pauli, S. (1998). Brain distortions in patients with primarily generalized tonic-clonic seizures. *Epilepsia* **39**, 364–370.

Sisodiya, S.M. and Free, S.L. (1997). Disproportion of cerebral surface areas and volumes in cerebral dysgenesis. MRI-based evidence for connectional abnormalities. *Brain* **120**, 271–281.

Sisodiya, S.M., Free, S.L., Stevens, J.M., Fish, D.R. and Shorvon, S.D. (1995). Widespread cerebral structural changes in patients with cortical dysgenesis and epilepsy. *Brain* **118**, 1039–1050.

Stevens, J.R. (1970). Focal abnormality in petit mal epilepsy – intracranial recordings and pathological findings. *Neurology* **20**, 1069–1076.

Stewart, L.F. and Dreifuss, F.E. (1967). 'Centrencephalic' seizure discharges in focal hemispheral lesions. *Arch Neurol* **17**, 60–68.

Swartz, B.E., Halgren, E., Simpkins, F. and Syndulko, K. (1994). Primary memory in patients with frontal and primary generalized epilepsy. *J Epilepsy* **7**, 232–241.

Swartz, B.E., Simpkins, F., Halgren, E. *et al.* (1996). Visual working memory in primary generalized epilepsy: an ¹⁸FDG PET study. *Neurology* **47**, 1203–1212.

Velasco, M., Velasco, F., Velasco, A.L., Luján, M. and del Mercado, J.V. (1989). Epileptiform EEG activities of the centromedian thalamic nuclei in patients with intractable partial motor, complex partial, and generalized seizures. *Epilepsia* **30**, 295–306.

Williams, D. (1953). A study of thalamic and cortical rhythms in petit mal. *Brain* **76**, 50–69.

Woermann, F.G., Sisodiya, S.M., Free, S.L. and Duncan, J.S. (1998a). Quantitative MRI in patients with idiopathic generalized epilepsy (IGE): evidence of widespread cerebral structural changes. *Brain* **121**, 1661–1667.

Woermann, F.G., Free, S.L., Koepp, M.J., Sisodiya, S.M. and Duncan, J.S. (1998b). Quantitative MRI in patients with juvenile myoclonic epilepsy (JME): an objective voxel-based comparison of structural imaging data [Abstract]. *Neuroimage* **7**, S502.

Juvenile Myoclonic Epilepsy: The Janz Syndrome
Edited by Bettina Schmitz and Thomas Sander
© 2000 Wrightson Biomedical Publishing Ltd

9

Positron Emission Tomography in Idiopathic Generalized Epilepsy: Imaging Beyond Structure

MATTHIAS J. KOEPP and JOHN S. DUNCAN

Institute of Neurology, National Hospital for Neurology and Neurosurgery, London, UK

Standard structural imaging with X-ray computerized tomography (CT) and magnetic resonance imaging (MRI) is normal in idiopathic generalized epilepsies (IGE), and positron emission tomography (PET) provides a potential means to advance our understanding of these conditions. PET allows tomographic delineation of cerebral structures and measurement of local tissue concentrations of injected radioactive tracers. PET can be performed with the subject in the resting state, or during or following a cognitive or motor task, the administration of a drug or the occurrence of a seizure. PET depends on the use of short half-life positron-emitting isotopes. The most commonly used isotopes are ^{15}O, ^{11}C, and ^{18}F which have half-lives of 2, 20 and 110 minutes respectively. Of these ^{15}O and ^{11}C are substituted for naturally occurring elements. The use of natural elements allows labelling of compounds for use *in vivo* without altering their biochemical properties or behaviour, which enables PET to image molecular pathways and pre- and postsynaptic binding sites.

In the field of IGE, PET has been used to study:

- regional cerebral glucose metabolism (rCMRglu) with ^{18}F-fluoro-2-deoxyglucose (^{18}F-FDG)
- regional cerebral blood flow (rCBF) with ^{15}O-H$_2$O
- receptor localization and kinetics of:
  μ-, k- and ∂-opiate receptors with ^{11}C-diprenorphine (DPN)
  central benzodiazepine receptors (cBZR) with ^{11}C-flumazenil (FMZ)

REGIONAL CEREBRAL GLUCOSE METABOLISM (rCMRglu) AND CEREBRAL BLOOD FLOW (rCBF)

The relationship between spike-wave activity and cerebral glucose utilization is not straightforward. In an autoradiographic study of cerebral glucose utilization in a rat model of spontaneous generalized absences, there was a widespread increase in cerebral glucose metabolism, compared with controls. However, a dose of ethosuximide that suppressed all spike-wave activity was not associated with a reduction of glucose metabolism (Nehlig et al., 1992). There have been three studies of glucose metabolism in IGE in humans. Interictal studies have been unremarkable; studies carried out when frequent absences were occurring have shown a diffuse increase in cerebral glucose metabolism of 30–300%, with greater increases being seen in children. Absence status, however, was associated with a reduction in cerebral glucose metabolism. There were no focal abnormalities and the rate of metabolism did not correlate with the amount of spike-wave activity (Engel et al., 1985; Theodore et al., 1985; Ochs et al., 1987).

Swartz et al. (1997) examined relative regional changes in FDG uptake during a visual working memory paradigm in patients with juvenile myoclonic epilepsy (JME). At rest, JME patients and controls could be discriminated by changes in the ventral premotor area, with relative decreases of glucose metabolism in JME patients. The working memory task appeared to enhance and expand these differences in the premotor and prefrontal areas. In the JME patients, unlike control subjects, increased activity was not found during the working memory task in the dorsolateral-prefrontal cortex, with the ventral premotor area being highly associated.

Regional cerebral blood flow (rCBF) has been assessed using PET and bolus injections of ^{15}O-labelled water and PET, achieving a temporal resolution of < 30 seconds and a spatial resolution of $8 \times 8 \times 4.3$ mm. Typical absences were precipitated with hyperventilation and the distribution of rCBF was compared when absences did and did not occur. During absences there was a global 15% increase in rCBF and, in addition, a focal 4–8% increase in blood flow to the thalamus. There were no focal increases in rCBF in the cortex and no focal decreases (Prevett et al., 1995a). Spike-wave activity in typical absences oscillates in thalamocortical circuits and the site of primary abnormality remains uncertain. The preferential increase in thalamic blood flow is evidence to the key role of this structure in the pathophysiology of absences in man, but does not clarify whether this is the result of converging activated thalamocortical pathways or reflects a primary thalamic process. No significant increases in thalamic blood flow were detected in the 30 seconds prior to generalized spike-wave activity on the EEG. A focal increase in blood flow developing five seconds before generalized spike-waves appeared would be most unlikely to be detected with this technique.

OPIATE RECEPTORS

Regional cerebral blood flow (rCBF) and rCMRglu reflect local synaptic activity and ^{15}O-H$_2$O PET activation studies have increased our understanding of the functional anatomy of the brain in health and disease. Neurotransmitters are responsible for mediating human neuronal activity and, until now, PET studies of specific ligands have largely been limited to quantitation of receptor binding and availability under resting conditions. Endogenous neurotransmitter release is a pivotal event in neuroregulation, but has been very difficult to study noninvasively *in vivo* in man (Morris *et al.*, 1995). Until 1993, PET studies of neurotransmitter release in humans concentrated on pharmacological manipulations and measured changes in receptor availability to radioligands (Dewey *et al.*, 1993).

Systemic administration of opioids tends to cause an increase in generalized spike-wave activity, in contrast to the anticonvulsant effect of endogenous opioids on generalized tonic-clonic seizures, suggesting that opioid transmission may have a role in the pathogenesis of absences (Frey and Voits, 1991). Diprenorphine is an opiate receptor antagonist with similar *in vivo* affinities for the mu, kappa and delta receptor subtypes. There was no significant difference in ^{11}C-diprenorphine binding between control subjects and patients with childhood and juvenile absence epilepsy, suggesting that there is no overall abnormality of opioid receptors in this condition (Prevett *et al.*, 1995a).

In a dynamic study, however, it was found that serial absences were associated with an acute 15–41% reduction in ^{11}C-diprenorphine binding to association areas of neocortex, with no effect on binding to thalamus, basal ganglia or cerebellum (Bartenstein *et al.*, 1993). The results implied release of endogenous opioids in the neocortex that displaced the injected radioligand from the receptor, thus reducing the amount of bound ^{11}C-diprenorphine. The results implied release of endogenous opioids in the neocortex that may have a role in the pathophysiology of typical absences. Further studies with subtype-specific ligands may provide information about the role of different opioid receptor subtypes in typical absences.

CENTRAL BENZODIAZEPINE RECEPTOR (cBZR)

Group analyses of interictal PET studies could provide information about underlying mechanisms or adaptive responses. Interictal FMZ studies have indeed revealed abnormalities of gamma-aminobutyric acid (GABA), the major inhibitory neurotransmitter in the central nervous system. Savic *et al.* (1990) reported a slight reduction in cortical binding of ^{11}C-FMZ to cBZR in a heterogeneous group of patients with generalized seizures, compared with the 'non-focus' areas of patients with partial seizures. It was subsequently reported that, compared with normal subjects, patients with primary generalized tonic-clonic seizures had an increased cBZR density in the cerebellar nuclei and decreased density in the thalamus (Savic *et al.*, 1994). Reliable identification of cerebellar nuclei is not easy on ^{11}C-FMZ PET images and these results have not been replicated. Prevett *et al.* (1995b) found no significant difference in ^{11}C-FMZ binding to cerebral cortex, thalamus or cerebellum between patients with childhood absence epilepsy (CAE) and juvenile absence epilepsy (JAE), not taking valproate (VPA), and control subjects. The volume of distribution of ^{11}C-FMZ, however, was 9% less in patients receiving VPA, suggesting that this drug may result in reduced number of available cBZR.

The aim of the authors' latest study was first to determine whether FMZ binding is normal in patients with IGE and secondly to determine the effect of VPA on this binding in a more powerful longitudinal design. Single ^{11}C-FMZ PET scans in 20 normal volunteers and paired scans in 10 patients with IGE were performed before and after the addition of VPA to their medication. Five of the 10 patients had a clear diagnosis of JME. To determine interindividual and, in paired scans, intraindividual differences of FMZ binding in cerebral cortex, cerebellum and thalamus, entirely objective methods of data analysis were used:

- ROI, defined by Gaussian clustering, which takes into account individual anatomical differences and minimizes partial volume effects by excluding white matter, to assess global differences in FMZ-V_d.
- Statistical parametric mapping (SPM), an entirely objective voxel-based analysis, to detect focal changes, either increases or decreases of FMZ binding.

FMZ binding was globally increased in cerebral cortex, thalamus and cerebellum by 12% in the patients compared with controls (Koepp *et al.*, 1997). This finding of an increased cBZR density in cerebral cortex, thalamus and cerebellum in IGE is of great interest in comparison with pathological reports of microdysgenesis in JME. Meencke and Janz (1984) reported that 14 of 15 patients with IGE had evidence of abnormal neuronal migration with an increase in dystopic neurons in the stratum moleculare, white matter, hippocampus and cerebellar cortex. Quantification of these changes has been difficult and these findings have been criticized (Lyon and Gastaut, 1985). However, although these changes can be seen in normal subjects, they were reported to be more severe and more frequent in patients with IGE than in control subjects (Meencke and Janz, 1985). Meencke (1985) found that neuron density of layer 1 in the frontal lobe in IGE patients was significantly increased compared with age-matched subjects. ^{11}C-FMZ acts as a marker of cBZ/GABA$_A$-receptor-bearing neurons and therefore the observed increase of available cBZR in patients with IGE may reflect increased numbers of neurons.

In addition to being a neuronal marker, FMZ is also a biochemical marker of the functional integrity of the GABAergic system. An increase in GABA$_A$ receptors in the thalamic relay nuclei could contribute to a tendency to absences, although GABA$_B$ receptors have a major role in this process. An upregulation of GABA$_A$ receptors in the cerebral cortex would not be a tenable primary explanation for cortical hyperexcitability, but could be an adaptive response or may perturb the functioning of thalamocortical circuits, facilitating synchronization of discharges.

It is not possible to be certain, at present, whether the observed increase of cBZ/GABA$_A$ receptors is due to an increase in neuronal density, is part of a functional pathogenic process underlying IGE, or is a secondary, adaptive phenomenon. Correlative quantitative neuropathology and autoradiographic studies are needed to resolve this issue.

Comparing the five patients with JME with the 20 control subjects the authors found, in addition to a generalized increased FMZ binding, accentuated focal increases bilaterally in the dorsolateral prefrontal cortex (DLPFC) and ventral premotor area (see Figure 1). These bi-frontal areas are close to those areas 45 and 46 in the medial and inferior frontal gyrus, where the most profound increases in neuronal density had been observed. These focal accentuations were not seen when comparing the five remaining IGE patients with 20 controls.

The mid-frontal areas could be related to the maximum spike negativity in absences previously shown to be at similar mid-frontal sites in topographical EEG analyses. However, these frontal changes were found both before and on VPA treatment in JME patients and did not seem to be related to the frequency of absences. The changes in the DLPFC could be the pathological substrate for the anecdotally reported behavioural disturbances in JME, which are reminiscent of a frontal lobe personality with emotional instability, lack of discipline and a tendency to jump from one place to another. These findings of abnormalities within the GABAergic system are very similar in location to the changes found in the FDG PET study by Swartz et al. (1997) described above. Together, these two PET studies suggest that patients with JME may suffer from cortical functional disorganization that affects both the epileptogenic potential and cognitive frontal lobe functioning.

Treatment with VPA did not change FMZ binding, neither did the concomitant reduction in seizures. The duration of VPA treatment was relatively short, 4–16 weeks, and only half of the patients were completely seizure-free at the time of the second scan. However, the cortical, but not thalamic, FMZ binding in the five treatment responders was reduced in four out of those five who became seizure-free. Since GABAergic neurons in

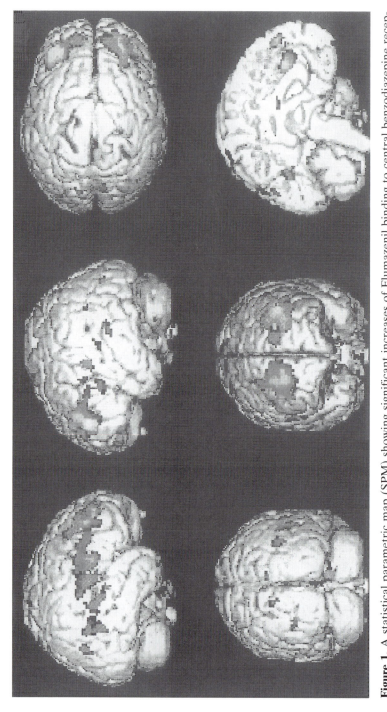

Figure 1. A statistical parametric map (SPM) showing significant increases of Flumazenil binding to central benzodiazepine receptors bilaterally in the dorsolateral prefrontal cortex of five patients with juvenile myoclonic epilepsy when compared to 20 healthy controls. These changes were not seen when comparing patients with childhood or juvenile absence epilepsy to controls.

different nuclei may play mutually counterposing roles, changes in $GABA_A$-receptor-related measures cannot be easily interpreted. GABA agonists exacerbate generalized spike-wave activity, benzodiazepines enhance the action of GABA at $GABA_A$ receptors and yet suppress absence seizures. The best explanation for this apparent paradox is that GABA has site-specific action: in the cerebral cortex GABA has predominantly inhibitory action, whereas in the thalamus enhancement of $GABA_A$ transmission increases spike-wave activity. The observed relative reduction or downregulation of FMZ binding back to normal levels in patients who became seizure free could then mean increased levels of cortical GABA.

A further theoretical possibility is that increased ^{11}C-FMZ binding may reflect decreased cBZR occupancy by endogenous ligands. There is evidence from animal experiments and *in vitro* studies for endogenous benzodiazepine-like substances (endozepines) (Rothstein *et al.*, 1992) implying that such compounds have a role in the neurochemical regulation of behaviour (Nutt *et al.*, 1990). Endozepines may have a modulatory role in the pathophysiology of seizures. Release of endozepines has been very difficult to study noninvasively. However, in an investigation of changes of ^{11}C-FMZ binding during and after hyperventilation-induced absences the authors did not find direct evidence for release of endozepines (Prevett *et al.*, 1995c). Cerebral binding of ^{11}C-FMZ was not affected by flurries of absences in any area of neocortex or the thalamus, implying that binding to this part of the $GABA_A$-BZR was not involved in the pathophysiology of absences.

CONCLUSIONS

- The primary site of abnormal spike-wave activity oscillating in thalamo-cortical circuits remains uncertain. The preferential increase in thalamic blood flow is evidence of the key role of this structure in the pathophysiology of absences, but does not clarify whether this is the result of converging activated thalamocortical pathways or whether it reflects a primary thalamic process.

- Using the novel PET method of ligand displacement the authors could show that release of endogenous opioids in the cortex also plays an important role in the pathophysiology of absences. Further studies with subtype-specific ligands are necessary to elucidate which receptor is responsible for what type of action, pro- or antiepileptic.

- It is not possible to be certain at present whether the observed increase of cortical $BZ/GABA_A$ receptors is due to an increase in neuronal density, microdysgenesis, is part of a functional pathogenetic process underlying IGE, or is a secondary, adaptive phenomenon reflecting cortical hyperexcitability.

• The authors' longitudinal study suggested that VPA does not have a significant direct effect on the numbers of cBZR available for binding.
Reduction of cortical FMZ binding following treatment with VPA in
patients who became seizure-free could be equivalent to rendering those
patients less susceptible to seizures, and consistent with the view that
absences are generalized inhibitory seizures.

FUTURE STUDIES

Further studies with specific ligands, especially for $GABA_B$ and excitatory
amino acid receptors, may provide information about the role of different
neuroreceptors, in the pathogenesis of absences. This could help to further
refine certain subgroups of JME and IGE patients in terms of receptor profile
'fingerprinting'. In this context it will be especially interesting to study
families with affected members and at-risk relatives in a longitudinal fashion.
The future of PET will be studies of receptors, drug-binding and treatment
response, and especially neurotransmitter activation studies. PET also has the
potential to image gene-expression. PET imaging of the neurochemistry of
behaviour and cognition can be readily applied, and it would be most interesting to see whether certain personality traits, neuropsychological profiles
and behaviours of patients with JME can be visualized and localized using
modern imaging techniques, which are looking beyond structure.

REFERENCES

Bartenstein, P.A., Duncan, J.S., Prevett, M.C. *et al.* (1993). Investigation of the opioid
    system in absence seizures with positron emission tomography. *J Neurol Neurosurg
    Psychiatry* **56**, 1295–1302.
Dewey, S.L., Smith, G.S., Logan, J. *et al.* (1993). Effects of central cholinergic block-
    ade on striatal dopamine release measured with positron emission tomography in
    normal human subjects. *Proc Natl Acad Sci U S A* **90**, 11816–11820.
Engel, J.J., Lubens, P., Kuhl, D.E. and Phelps, M.E. (1985). Local cerebral metabolic
    rate for glucose during petit mal absences. *Ann Neurol* **17**, 121–128.
Frey, H.H. and Voits, M. (1991). Effect of psychotropic agents on a model of absence
    epilepsy in rats. *Neuropharmacol* **30**, 651–656.
Koepp, M.J., Richardson, M.P., Brooks, D.J., Cunningham, V.J. and Duncan, J.S.
    (1997). Central benzodiazepine-$GABA_A$ receptors in idiopathic generalised
    epilepsy: an ^{11}C-flumazenil PET study. *Epilepsia* **38**, 1089–1097.
Lyon, G. and Gastaut, M. (1985). Considerations on the significance attributed to
    unusual cerebral findings recently described in eight patients with primary gener-
    alised epilepsy. *Epilepsia* **26**, 365–367.
Meencke, H.J. (1985). Neuron density in the molecular layer of frontal cortex in
    primary generalised epilepsy. *Epilepsia* **26**, 368–371.
Meencke, H.J. and Janz, D. (1984). Neuropathological findings in primary generalised
    epilepsy: a study of eight cases. *Epilepsia* **5**, 8–21.

Meencke, H.J. and Janz, D. (1985). The significance of microdysgenesis in primary generalised epilepsy: an answer to the consideration of Lyon and Gastaut. *Epilepsia* **26**, 368–371.

Morris, E.D., Fisher, R.E., Alpert, N.M., Rauch, S.L. and Fischman, A.J. (1995). *In vivo* imaging of neuromodulation using positron emission tomography: optimal ligand characteristics and task length for detection of activation. *Hum Brain Map* **3**, 35–55.

Nehlig, A., Vergnes, M., Marescaux, C. and Boyet, S. (1992). Mapping of cerebral energy metabolism in rats with genetic generalised nonconvulsive epilepsy. *J Neural Transm* **35** (suppl), 141–153.

Nutt, D.J., Glue, P. and Lawson, C.S.W. (1990). Flumazenil provocation of panic attacks. *Arch Psychol* **47**, 917–925.

Ochs, R.F., Gloor, P., Tyler, J.L. *et al.* (1987). Effect of generalised spike-and-wave discharge on glucose metabolism measured by positron emission tomography. *Ann Neurol* **21**, 458–464.

Prevett, M.C., Duncan, J.S., Jones, T., Fish, D.R. and Brooks, D.J. (1995a). Demonstration of thalamic activation during typical absence seizures using H_2O-^{15}O and PET. *Neurology* **45**, 1396–1402.

Prevett, M.C., Lammertsma, A.A., Brooks, D.J. *et al>* (1995b). Benzodiazepine-$GABA_A$ receptors in idiopathic generalised epilepsy measured with ^{11}C-flumazenil and positron emission tomography. *Epilepsia* **36**, 113–121.

Prevett, M.C., Lammertsma, A.A., Brooks, D.J., Cunningham, V.J., Fish, D.R. and Duncan, J.S. (1995c). Benzodiazepine-$GABA_A$ receptor binding during absence seizures. *Epilepsia* **6**, 592–599.

Rothstein, J.D., Garland, W., Puia, G., Guidotti, A., Weber, R.J. and Costa, E. (1992). Purification and characterization of naturally occurring benzodiazepine receptor ligands in rat and human brain. *J Neurochem* **58**, 2102–2115.

Savic, I., Pauli, S., Thorell, J.O. and Blomquist, G. (1994). *In vivo* demonstration of altered benzodiazepine receptor density in patients with generalised epilepsy. *J Neurol Neurosurg Psychiatry* **57**, 797–804.

Savic, I., Widen, L., Thorell, J.O. and Blomquist, G. (1994). Cortical benzodiazepine receptor binding in patients with generalised and partial epilepsy. *Epilepsia* **31**, 724–730.

Swartz, B.E., Simpkins, F., Halgren, E. *et al.* (1997). Visual working memory in primary generalized epilepsy: an ^{18}FDG-PET study. *Neurology* **47**, 1203–1212.

Theodore, W.H., Brooks, R., Margolin, R. *et al.* (1985). Positron emission tomography in generalised seizures. *Neurology* **35**, 684–690.

Juvenile Myoclonic Epilepsy: The Janz Syndrome
Edited by Bettina Schmitz and Thomas Sander
© 2000 Wrightson Biomedical Publishing Ltd

10

Cognitive and Personality Profiles in Patients with Juvenile Myoclonic Epilepsy

MICHAEL TRIMBLE

Institute of Neurology, London, UK

INTRODUCTION

The association between epilepsy and some kind of personality disorder has a long history. The literature of the nineteenth century, particularly in France and Germany, abounds with descriptions of personality changes in patients with epilepsy; these stem largely from physicians who were working in asylums, and patients with chronic epilepsy for which, in those times, there was virtually no treatment. The longstanding consequences of recurrent epileptic seizures led to a variety of presentations, from subtle alterations of personality to frank psychoses. Obviously, at this time, categorization of differing behaviour patterns, which became more popular towards the end of the century, and which dominated psychiatry in the twentieth century, were not available.

Interlinked with the concept of a personality change in epilepsy was the concept of hereditary degeneration, an interesting example of this thinking being provided by Turner (1907, p. 2), with the following description.

In early days the convulsion, or fit, was regarded as the sole element of importance in the clinical study of epilepsy: but in more recent years the psychical factor has come to be looked upon as of almost equal importance, and both are regarded as the manifestations of a predisposition associated with inheritance ... it is rare to find epileptics who do not present some form of mental obliquity ... the possession of which is a feature of their hereditary degenerative disposition ... the mental condition is not solely the consequence of seizures but is an expression of the same nervous constitution which gives rise to the convulsion.

This line of thinking was taken a further step forward, in the light of Freudian psychodynamics, in the early part of the twentieth century by writers such as Clarke (1923) who recognised pre-epileptic constitutions, and who went on to suggest that the seizure itself was some kind of psychological regressive or protective mechanism employed by an overstressed ego.

Thus, early on, two different concepts were being put forward. The first was that some kind of organic personality change occurred in people with epilepsy, consequent upon recurrent epileptic seizures and associated cerebral damage. The second was that patients with epilepsy were somehow constitutionally predisposed to a certain personality style which itself was predisposed to lead to seizures. The former view has led on to the concept of the interictal personality disorders associated with temporal lobe epilepsy. This was best summarized by Gibbs and Stamps (1953) when they noted that 'the patient's emotional reactions to his seizures, his family and to his social situation are less important determinants of psychiatric disorder than the site and type of the epileptic discharge'. The concept of a rather specific constellation of personality changes in temporal lobe epilepsy received further support from authors such as Gastaut *et al.* (1953) and then more recently Geschwind and colleagues (Waxman and Geschwind, 1975). They highlighted specifically changes in sexual behaviour, a deepening of both religious and mystical feelings, hypergraphia, and some kind of stickiness or viscosity of thinking, with patients showing a preoccupation for detail and excessive concerns over moral and ethical issues. Landolt (1960) had written about similar issues.

The profiles of other patients with other forms of epilepsy, however, have been little studied, although with particular reference to the syndrome of Janz, even his early descriptions suggested interesting personality variables which may be interlinked with his syndrome.

THE EARLY CONTRIBUTIONS

Janz, in a series of papers, described the clinical presentation of what is now referred to as Janz syndrome, or impulsive petit mal. The descriptions, initially based on a series of 47 patients, contained details of the seizures, electroencephalograms (EEGs) and personality profiles. Taking into account clinical observations, and also interviews with relatives, Janz and Christian (1994) commented in particular on the patients' behaviour concerning sleep. They noted that these patients awoke with difficulty in the morning, took some time to become fully conscious, and could remain 'sleep drugged' for even longer. All patients stressed that they required 'much sleep', but most of them apparently slept soundly. However, as a rule they were said to go to sleep late, and their sleep profile was thus one of late sleep and late awakening.

Janz and Christian thought that this sleep profile was constitutional, and not a secondary consequence of the epilepsy. They went on to describe the personality profile of these patients, which was contrary to 'typical epileptic behaviour', and their mental state was very often characterized by 'unsteadiness, lack of discipline, hedonism, and indifference towards their disease'.

All of their patients except one was of average intellectual ability, although none was particularly gifted. They commented that these patients tend to 'promise more than they can deliver', and on their 'pathological lack of ambition and endurance'. These features could lead to problems with treatment, patients tending to be noncompliant with medication, and often forgetting to attend outpatient visits.

To quote further, Janz and Christian said:

They often appeared self assured and bragging, the girls and women coquettish and seducing, but they only act decidedly mistruthfully and are timid, frightened and inhibited. Their labile feelings of self worth lead them to be both eager to help, to invite, to give, on the one hand and to be able to react in an exaggeratedly sensitive way on the other hand. Their mood changes rapidly and frequently. This makes their contact both charming and difficult. They are easy to encourage and to discourage, they are gullible and unreliable. Their suggestibility makes contacts easily but makes trust difficult. This personality profile plays along a scale from likeable nonchalance or timidity, through a psychasthenic syndrome to the extremes represented by sensitive or reckless psychopathy.

Further references to these personality types can be found in the paper by Tellenbach (1998) in which he describes the characteristic features of patients with Janz syndrome as 'impressionability, unreliability, instability, a tendency to extremes which is difficult to describe, a sentimental, sensitive personality continuously diverted by external events, whose development never matures into a harmonious personality'.

An early attempt to assess this personality style experimentally was that of Leder (1967, 1969) who compared the psychological profile of patients with *Aufwach* (awakening) epilepsy with patients with *Schlaf* (sleep) epilepsy using a number of subjective tests, mainly from the Rorschach or the Szondi batteries. They commented on the perseverative nature of the responses of the patients with sleep epilepsy and their enechetish constitution. The patients with Aufwach-epilepsy were referred to as 'extratensive' with a disturbed inner-outward relation and they were said to have an inflated 'Ichstörung'.

STUDIES USING NONSUBJECTIVE RATING SCALES

Two studies have examined in more detail the personality profile of patients with Janz syndrome. The first was that of Bech *et al.* (1977). They used the

Table 1. A comparison between patients with JME, TLE and diabetes of
psychopathology ratings (from Perini *et al.*, 1996).

	JME	*TLE*	*Diabetes*
No. of patients	18	20	20
SADS	22%	80%*	10%
Depression	16%	55%*	20%
BDI	9	18*	7
ANX (St)	38	47*	38
ANX (TR)	41*	52*	38

*Significant.

Marke–Nyman Inventory, a rating scale based upon the psychological
theories of Sjøbring. They gave the scale to 30 patients with JME, 29 with
psychomotor epilepsy, 30 with grand mal epilepsy, and 22 control patients
with Menière's disease. Essentially few differences were noted between the
groups although patients with JME were said to show low validity compared
with other groups.

Perini *et al.* (1996) compared 20 patients with temporal lobe epilepsy with
18 with Janz syndrome, 20 with diabetes and 20 normal controls on the SADS
(Schedule for Affective Disorders and Schizophrenia – a structured psychiatric interview) and rating scales of depression and anxiety. The results
showed (Table 1) significant differences between patients with temporal lobe
epilepsy and Janz syndrome, the former showing more abnormal profiles.
Indeed, the patients with Janz syndrome showed only one significant difference from controls by having high scores on a trait anxiety scale.

Only four patients with Janz syndrome met Research Diagnostic Criteria
for a psychiatric disorder, compared with 16 of the patients with temporal
lobe epilepsy. The diagnoses given were three minor depressions and one
generalized anxiety disorder.

COGNITIVE STUDIES

Janz, in his original descriptions, noted the EEG changes which were bilateral
and which often predominated frontally. While imaging studies tend to be
negative in patients with Janz syndrome the possibility that frontal lobe
functions may be compromised in the disorder has been tested by Devinski *et
al.* (1997). They took 16 patients with the syndrome, and excluded patients
with low scores on the Wechsler Intelligence Scale. They compared their data
on a number of frontal lobe tasks with 15 patients with temporal lobe
epilepsy, matched for IQ. The frontal tests used included motor function
(grooved peg board, finger oscillation and selected Luria tests of alternating

Table 2. Neurocognitive studies in JME (from Devinsky *et al.*, 1997), % abnormalities.

WCS (Wisconsin Card Sorting Test)	60
Category test	64
Luria sequences	67
STROOP	53
Trails	47
Pegboard	42
Mazes	33
Word association	21

sequences), psychomotor speed (trail-making test and the STROOP test), planning tasks (the Wechsler mazes), a verbal fluency task, and abstract reasoning and concept formation tasks such as the Wisconsin Card Sorting Test and the Booklet Categories Test.

The results from the patients with Janz syndrome were not homogeneous, and the percentage of patients impaired is given in Table 2. Significant differences between the group with Janz syndrome and the temporal lobe group were found for the trail-making test, part B, and the Wisconsin Card Sorting Test for categories and perseverative responses, the patients with the syndrome having the worse results.

Devinski *et al.* (1997) suggested that their results supported previous suggestions that patients with JME had normal IQs, but impaired performance on some frontal tasks. They commented on the differences between this profile of cognitive changes and that found in temporal lobe epilepsy.

Swartz *et al.* (1994) examined memory function in a group of nine patients with JME, a group of 15 patients with frontal lobe epilepsy, and a group of 15 normal controls. The key test was the delayed match to sample, which they refer to as a measure of a primary or working memory. The frontal lobe epilepsy group performed the worst, the JME group appearing intermediate between the controls and the frontal subjects.

Taken together, these data do suggest subtle but nonetheless real frontal impairments in people with Janz syndrome.

ON THE RELATIONSHIP OF JME TO FORCED NORMALIZATION

One of the factors that led Janz to his initial descriptions was studying the relationship of the epilepsies to the sleep–wake cycle. Janz made early observations that there were considerable differences between the epilepsies that presented with generalized tonic-clonic seizures occurring in sleep and those that occurred with awakening, the latter being frequently precipitated by external factors such as emotional and physical stress, excessive socialization, and lack of sleep. He noted that unusual lack of sleep, excess alcohol intake and early arousal seemed common precipitants for the seizures at the initial onset of the disorder, which continued during the clinical course of the syndrome. This appears to have led to an interesting debate about the relationship of different forms of epilepsy to sleep patterns. It seems that essentially the epilepsies on awakening came to be regarded as generalized epilepsies while those arising during sleep were likely to be focal epilepsies, probably temporal in origin. The differing relationship to sleep therefore not only applied to the pattern of the seizures, but also to the underlying neurophysiology and pathology, and also to the ensuing personality profiles.

Forced normalization, the phenomenon initially recognized by Landolt in the 1950s, described a concept whereby patients with successful therapy of their seizures with anticonvulsant drugs, would develop an acute behaviour change, which lasted for as long as the seizures were suppressed and was accompanied by a normalization of the previously abnormal EEG. The whole field has recently been reviewed in detail (Trimble and Schmitz, 1998), but one of the interesting debates that went on in the early papers on this subject was about the relationship between different forms of epilepsy and the developing alternative psychosis. Janz (1969, 1998) pointed out that Christian was the first person to describe forced normalization in a patient with awakening epilepsy, and how, following further observations, it was suggested that alternative psychoses were especially related to the 'rare combination of awakening epilepsies with psychomotor seizures'.

Tellenbach (1998) discussed this in more detail. Of his 12 cases, nine had grand mal epilepsy on awakening, and either the seizure disorder had started in this way, or there had been a preceding 'pyknoleptic prelude', which changed into this form of disorder, in four cases. None of the cases had epilepsy with seizures during sleep, but in seven of the 12 the course of the seizure disorder ended with a psychomotor epilepsy. He continued, 'it must be summarized that in the course of the epilepsy of our patients, a tendency from awakening epilepsy towards a psychomotor epilepsy cannot be overlooked'. This led on to the concept of 'secondary psychomotor epilepsy', which may have been one explanation for the developing paranoid psychosis following suppression of seizures.

Tellenbach then discussed possible neurophysiological explanations for both the behaviour changes and the EEG changes. Following therapy, patients were said to show 'a pervasive slowing which was out of character, sometimes reaching stupor and apathy, which was perceived by the patients in a negative way and limited their ability to express themselves'. Tellenbach went on to draw a parallel between the neurophysiological hypothesis of an excessive inhibitory activity, and the development of psychopathological symptoms, patients with epilepsy of awakening being particularly sensitive to this:

forced process of slowing down and of being constrained, as if being surrounded by a wall because of their personality traits of extraversion and impulsivity ... everything that threatens their stability will immediately and recklessly be expressed. It is clear that these patients are handicapped by the pathological slowing down arising from the interaction between medication and the brain. Because of this inability to create an affective balance they are increasingly less successful in keeping their stability in everyday life.

Tellenbach went on to note an important factor, which was the sleeplessness which could often be observed at this point in the clinical cycle, and effectively became a herald to the developing psychosis: 'The situation is accentuated by the already mentioned typology of patients with awakening epilepsy which is characterized by an affective lability, extraversion, infantilism, and sometimes antagonistic personality. This is why the psychotic syndromes of forced normalization express themselves in cases of awakening epilepsy in a dramatic way which fits the personality'. He observed that psychosocial conflicts often become more acute in the prepsychotic state, and how a vicious cycle of worsening behaviours and seizures develops.

CONCLUSIONS

The relationship between epilepsy and personality changes has had a long and considerably controversial background. The two main views that have been posited are either that patients have some kind of personality predisposition (constitutional or genetic) which leads them towards having seizures, or that the recurrent process of having seizures, with underlying neurological damage, slowly leads to change of personality which must be seen as a subtle organic brain syndrome. As time has progressed, within the twentieth century, we have seen the idea of susceptible personalities (a Freudian psychosomatic amalgam) lose favour to the more neurologically-based explanations, culminating in the descriptions of the temporal lobe interictal personality by Gastaut (1956) and by Waxman and Geschwind (1975).

When Janz originally described his syndrome, he noted particular personality characteristics, and suggested that these patients may bring with them an increased liability to develop the seizure disorder. This came in particular because of their altered sleep patterns, and somewhat reckless social behaviour. However, it also seemed to be the case that this personality style contributed to the progression of the syndrome, but itself was accentuated by the neurological consequences of the cerebral changes that were seen with the seizures of this syndrome. In a subgroup of patients, the development of a progressive psycho-organic syndrome occurred, often with psychotic features and a tendency to forced normalization, which was due to some kind of secondary development of a neurological focus in the temporal lobes.

Further, Janz and his followers have always been insistent upon the contribution of adverse psychosocial factors at the time of the development of these syndromes, thus combining the neurological, social and psychiatric aspects together in a more comprehensive way of understanding these syndromes than has been the *Zeitgeist* of epileptology in the last 40 years.

In spite of Janz's clear associations of his syndrome with personality changes, these have been consistently ignored by people who have reviewed or investigated the syndrome since then and, as this chapter reveals, only a very small number of studies have been undertaken in this area. They seem to support the view that patients with Janz syndrome are usually intellectually unimpaired, but may show some impairments on frontal lobe tasks. The latter may well be interlinked with the neurophysiological abnormalities seen in this form of epilepsy, with the emphasis on frontocentral EEG discharges.

There are too few studies which have attempted to objectify the personality characteristics of these patients to be of much help, except to conclude that these patients are clearly different in their behaviours from patients with temporal lobe epilepsy, in a way which Janz originally predicted.

REFERENCES

Bech, P., Petersen, K.K., Simmonsen, N. and Lund, M. (1977). Personality traits in epilepsy. In: Penry, J.K. (Ed.), *Epilepsy: the VIIIth International Symposium*. Raven Press, New York, pp. 257–263.

Clarke, L.P. (1923). The psychobiological concept of essential epilepsy. *J Nerv Ment Dis* **57**, 433–444.

Devinsky, O., Gershengorn, J., Brown, E. *et al.* (1997). Frontal functions in juvenile myoclonic epilepsy. *Neurol Neuropsychol Behav Neurol* **10**, 243–246.

Gastaut, H. (1956). La maladie de Vincent van Gogh. *Ann Medicopsychol* **114**, 196–238.

Gibbs, F.A. and Stamps, F.W. (1953). *Epilepsy Handbook*. Thomas Springfield.

Janz, D. (1969). *Die Epilepsien: spezielle Pathologie und Therapie*, Thieme, Stuttgart.

Janz, D. (1998). Episodic changes in mood and psychoses, In: Trimble, M.R. and Schmitz, B. (Eds). *Forced Normalization and Alternative Psychoses of Epilepsy*, Wrightson Biomedical, Petersfield.

Janz, D. and Christian, W. (1994). Impulsive petit mal. In: Malafosse, A., Genton, P., Hirsch, E. *et al* (Eds), *Idiopathic Generalised Epilepsies: Clinical Experimental and Genetic Aspects*. John Libbey, London, pp. 229–251.

Landolt, H. (1960). *Die Temporallappenepilepsie und ihre Psychopathologie*. Karger, Basel.

Leder, A. (1967). Zur Psychopathologie der Schlaf und Aufwachepilepsie (Eine psychodiagnostische Untersuchung). *Nervenarzt* **38**: 434–442.

Leder, A. (1969). *Aufwach Epilepsie*. Verlag Hans Huber, Bern, Germany.

Perini, G.I., Tosin, C., Carraro, C. *et al.* (1996). Interictal mood and personality disorders in temporal lobe epilepsy and juvenile myoclonic epilepsy. *J Neurol Neurosurg Psychiatry* **61**, 601–605.

Stauder, K.H. (1938). *Konstitution und Wesenänderung der Epileptiker*. Thieme, Leipzig.

Swartz, B.E., Halgren, E., Simpkins, F. and Syndulko, K. (1994). Primary memory in patients with frontal and primary generalised epilepsies. *J Epilepsy* **1**, 232–241.

Tellenbach, H. (1998). Epilepsy as a seizure disorder and as a psychosis: on alternative psychoses of a paranoid type with forced normalisation (Landolt) of the electroencephalogram of epileptics. Translated by L. Tebartz van Eltz. In: Trimble, M.R. and Schmitz, B. (Eds), *Forced Normalization and Alternative Psychoses of Epilepsy*. Wrightson Biomedical Publishing, Petersfield, pp. 49–66.

Trimble, M.R. and Schmitz, B. (1998). *Forced Normalization and Alternative Psychoses of Epilepsy*. Wrightson Biomedical Publishing, Petersfield.

Turner, A. (1907). *Epilepsy*. Macmillan, London.

Waxman, S.G. and Geschwind, N. (1975). The interictal behaviour syndromes of temporal lobe epilepsy. *Arch Gen Psychiatry* **32**, 1580–1586.

Juvenile Myoclonic Epilepsy: The Janz Syndrome
Edited by Bettina Schmitz and Thomas Sander
© 2000 Wrightson Biomedical Publishing Ltd

11

Response to Antiepileptic Drugs and the Rate of Relapse after Discontinuation in Juvenile Myoclonic Epilepsy

DIETER SCHMIDT

Epilepsy Research Group, Berlin, Germany

INTRODUCTION

A good response to antiepileptic drugs is usually associated with a low rate of relapse once the drug is withdrawn in patients in remission for several years (Schmidt and Gram, 1995). Why patients with juvenile myoclonic epilepsy (JME) who are generally thought to respond well to antiepileptic drugs (Commission on Classification and Terminology of the ILAE, 1989) appear to have such a high relapse rate remains unexplained. For example, Janz reported that a relapse may be expected in 75–100% of cases, even after many years of freedom from seizures, if the dosage is reduced or the drug discontinued (Janz *et al.*, 1983). One possible explanation could be that either the response of JME to valproate as the standard antiepileptic drug is not uniformly as good as has been suggested or the relapse rate has been overemphasized, or both. To test this hypothesis the evidence on the response to antiepileptic drugs, on seizure recurrence during drug treatment, and on relapse in patients with JME was critically re-examined.

METHODS AND DEFINITIONS

A favourable response has been defined in a recent population study on the prognosis of epilepsy in childhood as a reduction of 75–100% in the frequency of seizures within the first three months after the initiation of treatment (Commission on Classification and Terminology of the ILAE,1993). In the author's review the response within the first year of adequate treatment was studied. Any patient who is seizure-free for five years with or without medication at the time of ascertainment is generally considered to be in remission (Annegers *et al.*, 1979). Finally, one can assess whether patients had ever been in remission and whether they were still in remission at the time of the last follow-up or death. The difference in remission rates establishes the relapse rate. The definition of JME, a term introduced by Lund *et al.*, in 1976, followed that of the Commission of the International League Against Epilepsy (Commission on Classification and Terminology of the ILAE, 1989). Medline files were reviewed and specialist journals on epilepsy were hand-searched for publications on the outcome of drug treatment in JME.

RESPONSE TO TREATMENT AND SEIZURE RECURRENCE DURING TREATMENT

Surprisingly, the response to treatment of JME with valproate, or any other drug, has never been examined in a controlled trial (Schmidt, 1999). Instead, uncontrolled clinical observations are available which unfortunately cannot distinguish the observed outcome from effects unrelated to concurrent drug treatment. Clinical observations, in general, notoriously overestimate the effect of antiepileptic drugs (Schmidt, 1999). In patients with JME this is pertinent because confounding factors such as the precipitation of seizures through lack of sleep, often combined with alcohol consumption, are well established, and counselling patients on the danger of seizure precipitation and helping them to avoid it is established good clinical practice (Janz *et al.*, 1983). More recently, specific precipitatory factors that have been overlooked before were described in as many as 48% of patients in Japan (Inoue *et al.*, 1994). Wolf has recently described similar cases in Germany (Chapter 4 in this volume). Although never examined carefully, it has been suggested that avoiding nonspecific precipitation of seizures alone may be sufficient for seizure control in patients with early JME, especially those with myoclonic seizures alone. The effects of drug treatment may thus be confounded by concurrent, but unrelated, reduction in seizure precipitation. Conversely, transient exposure to precipitatory factors may lead to seizure recurrence despite continued drug treatment, as will be described in detail below. In addition, poor drug compliance may contribute to the recurrence of myoclonic and generalized tonic-clonic seizures (GTCS).

Another critical matter when evaluating the prognosis and long-term response to medication is the definition of the population studied. Ascertainment bias may limit the ability to generalize the findings from the patients studied to the syndrome as it occurs in the population (Cockerell *et al.*, 1997). JME is a syndrome that has not always been readily recognized in the past (Grünewald and Panayiotopoulos, 1993) and is therefore possibly underdiagnosed in large prospective population-based studies that started years ago. For example, a large UK study did not identify patients with myoclonic seizures and the patients are presumably included in the mixed generalized seizure heading (Cockerell *et al.*, 1997). In an earlier landmark study on remission and relapse, Annegers *et al.*, (1979) included 33 patients with myoclonic seizures. However, the course of these patients is not separately shown. As a consequence, no conclusions can be drawn from these otherwise very valuable data regarding specific syndromes such as JME which are rare at the population level. Furthermore, it is pertinent that most studies on the response of JME to antiepileptic drugs and the relapse after discontinuation in patients who had become seizure-free are hospital- and clinic-based and often involve patients who had been unsuccessfully treated for a long time before referral (Franzen, 1988; Delgado-Escueta and Enrile-Bacsal, 1994). With these methodological caveats the best clinical evidence is reviewed.

Based on uncontrolled studies, cessation of seizures is seen in three of four patients with JME receiving valproate. The percentage range is 33–100% (Table 1). In some, but not all, reports, recurrences of seizures during treatment are described. Seizure recurrence was associated with seizure-provoking lifestyle in patients with poor seizure control in as few as 7% (Delgado-

Table 1. Response to valproate (VPA) and recurrence of seizures during treatment in patients with JME.

Patients in remission	Seizure recurrence	Authors	Comment
19/30 (41%)	n.d.	Sharpe and Buchanan, 1995	VPA alone
37/49 (75%)	n.d.	Janz *et al.*, 1983	VPA alone or in combination; two-year remission; newly treated and inadequately pretreated patients
18/43 (41%)	n.d.	Kleveland and Engelsen, 1998	VPA alone; one-year remission
65/76 (88%)	n.d.	Atakli *et al.*,1998	VPA alone; two-year remission
32/40 (78%)	7%	Delgado-Escueta and Enrile-Bacsal, 1984	VPA alone or in combination; two-year remission
29/29 (100%)	14%	Franzen, 1988	VPA alone; after 3 years of treatment; newly treated and inadequately pretreated patients
43/50 (86%)	50%	Penry *et al.*, 1989	VPA mostly alone; one-year remission
42/50 (84%)	23%	Obeid and Panayiotopoulos, 1989	VPA alone or in combination; 6 months' remission
18/22 (82%)	n.d.	Bourgeois *et al.*, 1987	VPA alone; 9 months' treatment; generalized myoclonic seizures
2/6 (33%)	n.d.	Bruni *et al.*, 1980	VPA alone; EEG monitoring
Total 336/440 (76%)			

n.d., not described.

Escueta and Enrile-Bacsal, 1984) and as many as 50%. In the study where 25 patients (50%) reported recurrences during drug treatment due to precipitatory factors such as fatigue, noncompliance, sleep deprivation and alcohol consumption 12 patients had one recurrence, seven had two recurrences, three patients had three recurrences, two had two, and one patient had 11 recurrences. Previously untreated patients or those with myoclonic seizures alone were not described, if present (Penry *et al.*, 1989). In the experience of Reutens and Berkovic (1995) myoclonic seizures occur in response to precipitating factors such as sleep deprivation in about half the patients despite antiepileptic treatment. One study reported precipitatory factors in as many as 86% of patients (Atakli *et al.*, 1998). In one series where 44 patients (88%) with JME became seizure-free, mild myoclonic jerking continued in 10, particularly after sleep deprivation (Obeid and Panayiotopoulos, 1989). Finally, in a study of clonazepam, 11 of 12 patients with myoclonic seizures with or without tonic-clonic seizures became seizure-free for one year (Nanda *et al.*, 1977) and recent experience with lamotrigine has also been successful (Genton, Chapter 3 in this volume).

Little is known about the prognosis of patients with JME who have never been treated with antiepileptic drugs. The exception is a Norwegian study of 43 patients, where 7% were seizure-free without medication (Kleveland and Engelsen, 1998). Three of four relatives of patients with JME with jerks only had a spontaneous remission without any drug treatment (Jain *et al.*, 1997). The authors suggest that patients with myoclonic jerks only are a subgroup of JME, where jerks may remit spontaneously. Not surprisingly, patients having only myoclonic seizures may be a particularly easily treated subgroup of JME. In a report from India, 15 of 161 patients (9%) with JME having only myoclonic seizures were analysed. Nine probands and two relatives with only myoclonic jerks were treated with antiepileptic drugs. Myoclonic jerks alone, without GTCS and absence seizures occurred in 7–17% (Asconapé and Penry, 1984; Janz 1969; Penry *et al.*, 1989). The authors suggest that these percentages may be underestimated, because myoclonic jerks may be mild, being misinterpreted as early-morning clumsiness or nervousness. Three patients with previously untreated myoclonic seizures alone became seizure-free when clonazepam was added. However, one patient developed GTCS after the addition of clonazepam (Obeid and Panayiotopoulos, 1989). Finally, and perhaps surprisingly, the impact of training patients to avoid precipitation without treating them with antiepileptic drugs at the same time has never been evaluated.

In contrast to the good response to treatment described above, a number of reports undermine the conventional wisdom that JME is invariably associated with a good response to drug treatment. In the study by Franzen (1988) all 29 patients eventually became seizure-free. However, the data suggest that after three and five years of treatment only 62%, and 31% remained seizure-free while on medication. It should be noted that 60% of the patients were previously treated, presumably unsuccessfully, before being seen in a university referral centre. In a survey by Covanis *et al.*, (1982) 31 of 45 previously refractory patients (70%) with myoclonic seizure in adolescence, most likely JME, became seizure-free with valproate, while the others either showed no reaction on monotherapy or required a second drug. In a careful EEG-monitored study of six patients with myoclonic seizures only two were seizure-free and three had at least a 75% reduction after one year of treatment with valproate; one patient discontinued the drug (Bruni *et al.*, 1980). In the study by Asconapé and Penry, no more than six of 12 patients with JME became seizure-free, including two patients with myoclonic seizures only. Three patients showed a reduction and three patients needed a second drug added to valproate. One of the three patients had focal EEG features, one had atypical absence seizures, and one patient continued to have frequent myoclonic jerks and GTCS, despite effective levels of valproate alone or in combination with carbamazepine. This patient had auditory precipitation, a finding not previously described in patients with JME. In patients with precipitation-induced seizures, the response to drug treatment of JME may not be uniformly good. Response to antiepileptic drugs was assessed in 104 patients with JME. While 49 of 71 JME patients (69%) without reflex seizures were free from seizures for three years, only five of 17 patients (29%) with incidental and five of 16 patients (31%) with predominantly reflex triggering were free from seizures (Inoue *et al.*, 1994). This important study identified a difficult-to-treat subgroup of patients with induced JME that had been largely overlooked before. In a larger series of more than 200 patients, precipitatory factors were found to exist in as many as 29% of patients with JME (Inoue, Chapter 7 in this volume). Twenty-five patients with praxis-induced JME were treated adequately and 13 were found to be drug-resistant. The specific precipitatory factors included ideation or execution of complicated movements, sequential processing, such as playing games, complicated finger movements, drawing and writing. In addition, concentration or attention associated with these activities may contribute to the precipitation (Inoue *et al.*, 1994, and Chapter 7 in this volume). Precipitation of myoclonic seizures may possibly be related to a transiently decreased cortical inhibition of the motor cortex. The hypothesis was tested by magnetic brain stimulation. The absence of motor evoked potentials (MEPs) suppression and a progressive amplitude increase of MEPs was found in two patients with JME (Caramia *et al.*, 1996). Further studies are pertinent.

IS THE RESPONSE TO APPROPRIATE DRUGS UNIFORMLY GOOD IN JME?

The current international classification of epilepsies and syndromes curtly states that the response to appropriate drugs is good (Commission on

Classification and Terminology of the ILAE, 1989). Although most patients with JME respond well initially to drug treatment, e.g. with valproate, and in fact some patients with myoclonic seizures alone may not even need drug treatment, perhaps as many as 50% seen in hospital- and clinic-based series have seizure recurrences while under drug treatment, thus undermining the notion that all patients with JME have a good response to antiepileptic drugs. In fact, no controlled drug trials exist on the treatment of JME which could distinguish between the specific effects of drugs and concurrent reduction of precipitation unrelated to drug treatment. The role of training patients in how to avoid seizure precipitants is probably underutilized. Since as many as 50% of patients may have seizure recurrences while being treated with drugs, it is not surprising that relapse of seizures following the discontinuation of medication may be high in hospital- and clinic-based series.

SEIZURE RELAPSE AFTER DISCONTINUATION OF TREATMENT IN SEIZURE-FREE PATIENTS

In several small hospital- and clinic-based series of patients with often inadequately pre-treated JME, the rate of relapse following discontinuation of medication in remission for mostly two years has consistently been over 90% (Table 2). In a recent prospective study on relapse following discontinuation of antiepileptic drugs, 264 children with epilepsy who were seizure-free for 2.9 years were followed for a mean of 58 months to ascertain whether seizures occurred (Shinnar et al., 1994). Only four patients with JME were included and all four relapsed. In a landmark study of antiepileptic drug withdrawal in patients in remission, a history of myoclonic seizures was associated with a higher risk of seizure recurrence with a relative risk of 1.60 (95% confidence interval 0.98–2.60). It should be noted, however, that in the group of patients with myoclonic seizures alone (grouped together with simple or complex absences without tonic-clonic seizures) only nine of 1013 patients were randomized. The authors acknowledge that patients with JME were probably underdiagnosed; however, they found that patients with myoclonic seizures and GTCS were present in the trial although their actual number was not stated (MRC, 1991). In six previously inadequately treated patients who had finally become seizure-free with valproate alone for two years, myoclonic seizures or tonic-clonic seizures returned in all patients when valproate was withdrawn. However, no mention is made of poor compliance or seizure-provoking incidents such as staying up at night, although seizure recurrences while on medication due to precipitation were noted (Delgado-Escueta and Enrile-Bacsal,1984). In a larger series of 66 cases, nine of 11 patients relapsed after discontinuation of medication (Panayiotopoulos et al., 1994), six developed GTCS (one and three weeks and one, two, 12, and 16 months after

Table 2. Rate of relapse in patients with JME in remission following discontinuation of medication.

Rate of relapse	Authors	Comments
34/37 (91%)	Janz *et al.*, 1983	Discontinuation of VPA and other antiepileptic drugs in patients with myoclonic seizures and GTCS; after two-year remission, role of precipitatory factors not discussed
4/16 (25%)	Janz *et al.*, 1983	As above but only patients with myoclonic seizures or absence seizures alone
4/4 (100%)	Shinnar *et al.*, 1994	Discontinuation of antiepileptic drugs after 2.9 years of remission and 58 months of follow-up; precipitation not discusssed
9/11 (90%)	Panayiotopoulos *et al.*, 1994	One-year follow-up; precipitation in 93% of total series of 66 patients
6/6 (100%)	Delgado-Escueta and Enrile-Bacsal, 1984	Discontinuation of VPA; two-year remission; precipitation not discussed

VPA, valproate; GTCS, generalized tonic-clonic seizures.

discontinuation), one had myoclonic status (after two weeks), one had absence status (after three weeks), and one had a relapse of violent myoclonic jerks. The authors note that 93 % of their 66 patients had precipitating factors including sleep deprivation (89.5%), fatigue (73.7%), photosensitivity (36.8%), television and video games (8.8%), menstruation (24.1% of women), mental concentration (22.8%), and stress (12.3%). The authors commented further that absence seizures in patients with JME may sometimes be precipitated by concentration or excitement, but in general the absence seizures were not as sensitive to other factors that provoke myoclonic jerks and GTCS. It was further noted that it is rare for patients to present with JME after the age of 40 years, implying a decline in seizure susceptibility after the fourth decade.

The available evidence suggesting a high relapse rate of over 90% is difficult to interpret since the ascertainment-bias discussed above also applies to the study of relapse. If easy-to-treat patients, e.g. patients without precipitation of seizures, may be seen less often in hospital and clinics where in turn difficult-to-treat patients are primarily referred, population studies are needed to examine the long-term prognosis of JME. An example is the subgroup of patients with myoclonic seizures alone which may make up to as many as 17% of patients with JME, as discussed earlier. Patients with myoclonic seizures alone may have a much more favourable prognosis following discontinuation of medication. In a retrospective survey of case notes, Janz *et al.*, (1983) reported that 91% of 49 patients with JME having had myoclonic seizures and GTCS suffered a relapse when the medication was withdrawn. However, when patients with myoclonic seizures alone were assessed, the authors decided to include them in a group together with patients with absence seizures only, in which 84% became seizure-free and the relapse rate was a mere 25% (Table 2). Although the study may be criticized because the type of medication was not given and the impact of precipitatory factors was not discussed, the low relapse rate in patients with myoclonic seizures alone in contrast to patients with GTCS and myoclonic seizures is noteworthy. Furthermore, the relapse rate may possibly be lower in patients with JME who are not susceptible to seizure precipitation. The percentage of JME patients with or without seizure precipitation in the population is not known. In addition, JME is a relatively rare syndrome in the population; estimates range from 2 to 4 %. In large, population-based studies that started many years ago JME may have been underdiagnosed, as the authors concede (MRC, 1991, Cockerell *et al.*, 1997) and precipitation of seizures could not be analysed. Finally, precipitation of seizures in patients with JME may be age-related and decline when patients enter the third or fourth decade. This may perhaps explain why elderly patients with JME appear to be uncommon in epilepsy clinics (Genton, Chapter 3 in this volume).

HOW GOOD IS THE EVIDENCE FOR A UNIFORMLY HIGH RELAPSE RATE FOLLOWING DISCONTINUATION IN JME?

The high rate of relapse reported for referrals with previously inadequately treated patients may be due, at least in part, to uncorrected ascertainment bias. A likely explanation is that patients with precipitatory factors and those with myoclonic seizures and associated tonic-clonic seizures may be overrepresented. The ascertainment bias makes it difficult to generalize these findings to the patients with JME in the general population. This is not entirely an academic question but has grave implications for patient management. Based on the evidence reviewed above, lifelong anticonvulsant treatment is usually considered necessary in patients with JME, and withdrawal of medication in well controlled patients may precipitate seizures and status epilepticus. However, in patients with very infrequent seizures, Grünewald and Panayiotopoulos (1993) recently suggested that it may be safe to reduce the amount of medication, especially after the fourth decade of life, accepting that relapses are possible months or years after withdrawal. The present author might add that previously untreated patients who easily become seizure-free on valproate and learn how to avoid a seizure recurrence can be withdrawn safely. Finally, we should examine whether we are overtreating patients who can manage seizure control without medication. This is something that patients with JME have constantly told physicians, and some of us, including the author, may have not been listening. Careful studies of the role of individual seizure precipitation are pertinent and may change our view on the response of patients with JME to antiepileptic drugs, the rate of remission with or without drugs, and the rate of relapse in those in remission.

CONCLUSIONS

The main conclusion is that both the response to antiepileptic drugs and the rate of relapse have been determined by retrospective studies of biased cohorts, and that the uniformity *per se* of JME as an epileptic syndrome may be, at least in part, a result of selection bias. More specifically, the observations of a uniformly good response of patients with JME to antiepileptic drugs can no longer be upheld. While patients with myoclonic seizures alone or those who learn to control individual seizure precipitants may enter remission spontaneously, many patients in hospital- and clinic-based series have seizure recurrences while being treated, mainly due to precipitation of attacks and perhaps poor drug compliance. As many as 50% of clinic-based patients with JME may be susceptible to nonspecific and specific precipitation. In fact, precipitation and spontaneous remission are important confounding factors for the evaluation of the response to antiepileptic drugs. Controlled studies are needed. Furthermore, experimental models of JME and *in-vivo* studies in patients are needed in order to better understand the pathophysiology and precipitation of generalized myoclonic seizures. The prognosis of JME, with or without medication, needs to be examined in large, population-based prospective studies.

REFERENCES

Annegers, J.F., Hauser, W.A. and Elveback, L.R. (1979). Remission of seizures and relapse in patients with epilepsy. *Epilepsia* **20**, 729–737.

Asconapé, J. and Penry, J.K. (1984). Some clinical and EEG aspects of benign juvenile myoclonic epilepsy. *Epilepsia* **25**, 108–114.

Atakli, D., Sözüer, D., Atay, T., Baybas, S. and Arpaci, B. (1998). Misdiagnosis and treatment in juvenile myoclonic epilepsy. *Seizure* **7**, 63–66.

Bourgeois, B., Beaumanoir, B., Blajev, B. *et al.* (Collaborative Study Group) (1987). Monotherapy with valproate in primary generalized epilepsies. *Epilepsia* **28** (suppl. 2), 8–11.

Bruni, J., Wilder, B.J., Bauman, A.W. and Willmore, L.J. (1980). Clinical efficacy and long-term effects of valproic acid therapy on spike-and-wave discharges. *Neurology* **30**, 42–46.

Caramia, M.D., Gigli, G., Iani, C. *et al.* (1996). Distinguishing forms of generalized epilepsy using magnetic brain stimulation. *Electroencephalogr Clin Neurophysiol* **98**, 14–19.

Cockerell, O.C., Johnson, A.L., Sander, J.W.A.S. and Shorvon, S.D. (1997). Prognosis of epilepsy: a review and further analysis of the first nine years of the British national general practice study of epilepsy, a prospective population-based study. *Epilepsia* **38**, 31–46.

Commission on Classification and Terminology of the International League Against Epilepsy (1989). Proposal for revised classification of epilepsies and epileptic syndromes. *Epilepsia* **30**, 389–399.

Commission on Epidemiology and Prognosis, International League Against Epilepsy (1993). Guidelines for epidemiologic studies on epilepsy. *Epilepsia* **34**, 592–596.

Covanis, A., Gupta, A.K. and Jeavons, P.M. (1982). Sodium valproate: monotherapy and polytherapy. *Epilepsia* **23**, 693–720.

Delgado-Escueta, A.V. and Enrile-Bacsal, F. (1984). Juvenile myoclonic epilepsy of Janz. *Neurology* **34**, 285–294.

Franzen, S. (1988). Die medikamentöse Therapie der Epilepsien mit Impulsiv Petit Mal [Thesis]. Free University, Berlin.

Grünewald, R.A. and Panayiotopoulos, C.P. (1993). Juvenile myoclonic epilepsy. A review. *Arch Neurol* **50**, 594–598.

Inoue, Y., Seino, M., Kubota, H., Yamakaku, K., Tanaka, M. and Yagi, K. (1994). Epilepsy with praxis-induced seizures. In: Wolf, P. (Ed.), *Epileptic Seizures and Syndromes*. John Libbey, London, pp. 81–91.

Jain, S., Padma, M.V. and Maheshwari, M.C. (1997). Occurrence of only myoclonic jerks in juvenile myoclonic epilepsy. *Acta Neurol Scand* **95**, 263–267.

Janz, D. (1969). *Die Epilepsien: Spezielle Pathologie und Therapie*. Thieme Verlag, Stuttgart.

Janz, D. (1985). Epilepsy with impulsive petit mal (juvenile myoclonic epilepsy). *Acta Neurol Scand* **72**, 339–359.

Janz, D., Kern, A., Mössinger, H.-J. and Puhlmann, U. (1983). Rückfall-Prognose nach Reduktion der Medikamente bei Epilepsiebehandlung. *Nervenarzt* **54**, 525–529.

Kleveland, G. and Engelsen, B.A. (1998). Juvenile myoclonic epilepsy: clinical characteristics, treatment and prognosis in a Norwegian population of patients. *Seizure* **7**, 31–38.

Lund, M., Reintoft, H. and Simonsen, N. (1976). Eine kontrollierte soziologische und psychologische Untersuchung von Patienten mit juveniler myoklonischer Epilepsie. *Nervenarzt* **47**, 708–712.

Medical Research Council Antiepileptic Drug Withdrawal Study Group (1991). Randomised study of antiepileptic drug withdrawal in patients in remission. *Lancet* **337**, 1175–1180.

Nanda, R.N., Johnson, R.H., Keogh, H.J., Lambie, D.G. and Melville, I.D. (1977). Treatment of epilepsy with clonazepam and its effect on other anticonvulsants. *J Neurol Neurosurg Psychiatry* **40**, 538–543.

Obeid, T. and Panayiotopoulos, C.P. (1989). Clonazepam in juvenile myoclonic epilepsy. *Epilepsia* **30**, 603–606.

Panayiotopoulos, C.P., Obeid, T. and Tahan, A.R. (1994). Juvenile myoclonic epilepsy: a 5-year prospective study. *Epilepsia* **35**, 285–296

Penry, J.K., Dean, J.C. and Riela, A.R. (1989). Juvenile myoclonic epilepsy: long-term response to therapy. *Epilepsia* **30**, (suppl 4), 19–23.

Reutens, D.C. and Berkovic, S.F. (1995). Idiopathic generalized epilepsy of adolescence: are the syndromes clinically distinct? *Neurology* **45**, 1469–1476.

Schmidt, D. (1999). *Drug trials in epilepsy*. Martin Dunitz, London.

Schmidt, D. and Gram, L. (1995). Monotherapy versus polytherapy in epilepsy: a reappraisal. *CNS Drugs* **3**, 194–208.

Sharpe, C. and Buchanan, N. (1995). Juvenile myoclonic epilepsy: Diagnosis, management and outcome. *Med J Aust* **162**, 133–134.

Shinnar, S., Berg, A.T., Moshé, S.L. *et al.* (1994). Discontinuing antiepileptic drugs in children with epilepsy: a prospective study. *Ann Neurol* **35**, 534–545.

12

Maternal Use of Valproate during Pregnancy: Risk of Major Malformations and Brain Disorders

SABINE KOCH,[a] KARL TITZE,[b] SILVIA TREUTER,[b] MICHAEL SCHRÖDER,[c]
RALF B. ZIMMERMANN,[c] HANS-CHRISTOPH STEINHAUSEN,[d] HEINZ
NAU,[e] ULRIKE LEHMKUHL[b] and HELLGARD RAUH[f]

[a]*Rehabilitationsklinik für Kinder und Jugendliche, Kartzow-Beelitz in Beelitz-
Heilstätten, Germany*
[b]*Department of Child and Adolescent Psychiatry,
Psychosomatic Medicine and Psychotherapy and*
[c]*Department of Neurology, Charité Medical Faculty, Virchow Campus,
Humboldt University of Berlin, Germany*
[d]*Department of Child and Adolescent Psychiatry, University of Zürich, Switzerland*
[e]*Department of Food Toxicology, College of Veterinary Medicine,
Hannover, Germany*
[f]*Institute for Psychology, University of Potsdam, Germany*

INTRODUCTION

Seizures in juvenile myoclonic epilepsy are effectively controlled by valproic acid (VPA). VPA was also a generally accepted treatment for pregnant women with juvenile myoclonic epilepsy and other epilepsies characterized by primary generalized seizures. Since 1976, the authors' collaborative, prospective and longitudinal study on 'Epilepsy, Pregnancy and the Child', initiated in Berlin by H. Helge, D. Janz, H. Neubert and H.-C. Steinhausen (project co-ordinators), has aimed to detect potential teratogenic effects of prenatal drug exposure on the offspring of epileptic mothers. At the beginning of the study teratogenic effects of VPA on the human were not known and not expected. The first publication of clinical data from the Berlin study did not document a correlation of infant/fetal malformation with exposure to VPA (Nau *et al.*, 1981a). In a clinical study conducted at the same time in the Netherlands (Lindhout *et al.*, 1982), VPA as part of polytherapy was suspected to be terato-genic. In 1982 data of an epidemiological study in France indicated that women who were treated for epilepsy with VPA had an unexpected increase in births of children with spina bifida aperta (Robert and Gibaud, 1982). The Dutch study group subsequently also reported an increased risk of fetal malformations due to VPA exposure (Lindhout and Meinardi, 1984). By 1982 VPA was highly suspected being a teratogenic agent

Dosages of VPA for pregnant women in the Berlin study were about 10 mg/kg bodyweight in the years from 1977 to 1980 but were raised to 20–30 mg/kg bodyweight in the years from 1981 to 1983. Subsequently the paediatricians in the Berlin study observed differences in newborns who had been exposed to VPA in contrast to neonates exposed to other antiepileptic drugs, such as phenobarbitone, primidone, or phenytoin. VPA-exposed neonates had appropriate weight, length, and head circumference at birth, which was unusual in the neonates exposed to other drugs. However, they also had typical minor facial anomalies, such as a small mouth and nose, frontal bossing of the forehead, and wide epicanthic distance. Their fingers and toes were unusually long. One child had a major malformation of a ductus arteriosus apertus which closed spontaneously in the first year. In 1981 and 1983 three children were born with major malformations. One child suffered from a premature closing of the frontal suture, the second from a dysplasia of the sternum combined with hypoplasia of the first ribs. The last child was born with a lumbar spina bifida aperta and additional multiple malformations of the brain, the skeleton, the heart, and the kidney. These three children with major malformations also displayed the same specific minor anomalies that were observed in the VPA-exposed neonates without major malformations, though in much higher numbers (Jäger-Roman *et al.*, 1986). Their mothers had received the highest doses of VPA, up to 2000 mg/day, equaling 31 mg/kg bodyweight. Blood concentrations in these three mothers were above 100 μg/ml.

VPA appeared to be specifically teratogenic for neural tube defects. This suspicion was confirmed by Omzigt *et al.* (1992) in The Netherlands. Between 1985 and 1990, five out of 92 (5.4%) fetuses/neonates who had been exposed to VPA suffered a lumbosacral spina bifida aperta. The question is whether children who were prenatally exposed to VPA in varying dosages will be prone to additional and more discrete damage of the neuroepithelium, damage that will become evident only as functional disorders of the brain at preschool and school age. Teratogenic action on the developing fetal brain may result in malformations in the first trimester; in the second and third trimesters it will possibly result in functional disorders of the brain. It would be possible to follow up on these original study infants into preschool age and even adolescence.

SAMPLE AND DESIGN

The mothers with VPA treatment were a subgroup of a larger sample of pregnant women who entered the longitudinal prospective and controlled study between 1977 and 1983. The total group comprised 116 children of epileptic mothers with and 25 without therapy during pregnancy, 22 children of epileptic fathers, and an equal number of control children, matched to the risk group for parity and age of the mother, family social status, and maternal nicotine consumption (Steinhausen et al., 1994). Data from the 15 mother–child pairs with VPA as a monotherapy during pregnancy were drawn from the total sample for this analysis. With regard to sociodemographic criteria, this subsample did not differ either from the total group of epileptic mothers or from the control group.

Maternal epilepsy was classified according to the revised guidelines of the Commission on Classification and Terminology of the International League Against Epilepsy (1989) by Beck-Mannagetta. For study purposes the present authors simplified this classification. Drug dosage was measured relative to maternal bodyweight in the first trimester of pregnancy (mg/kg). Plasma concentrations of VPA were operationalized as the peak level measured all over pregnancy (in μg/ml).

The clinical-neurological examination of the infant at six months comprised 49 items. The number of items for each child assessed as nonoptimal during the examination is referred to here as the neurological measure. At six years and in adolescence, mild (MND1) and more pronounced minor neurological dysfunction (MND2) were determined with Touwen's scheme (1979) for neurological examination.

The children's intellectual ability was assessed with the Hannover–Wechsler Intelligence Test for preschool age (HAWIVA, Eggert, 1975), the German adaptation of the Wechsler Preschool and Primary School Scale of Intelligence (WPPSI), and during school age with the revised Hamburg Wechsler Intelligence Test for Children (HAWIK-R, Tewes, 1983), the German adaptation of the Wechsler Intelligence Scale for Children – Revised (WISC-R). Participants older than 14 years were tested with the revised Hamburg Wechsler Intelligence Test for Adults (HAWIE-E, Tewes, 1991), the German adaptation of the Wechsler Adult Intelligence Scale – Revised (WAIS-R). The examiner (K. Titze) was unaware of the child`s group classification.

Mental and behavioural disorders were diagnosed and classified according to the International Classification of Diagnoses (WHO, 1993). The examiner (S. Treuter) was trained in child psychiatry and unaware of the child's kind of prenatal drug exposure and the mother's medical history. The same was true for the electroencephalogram (EEG) scorers. The EEGs were inspected visually and coded by two trained neurologists (M. Schröder, R.B. Zimmermann) with the help of a coding manual. Specific scores were given for type, strength, and localization of background rhythm, for diffuse and focal slowing, and for epileptic discharges. Increased activity was separately coded for type, strength, localization, stimulus, and generality.

Table 1. Maternal and children's clinical data.

	Maternal data						Children's data								
Child no.	Year of birth	Seizure type	Grand mal during pregnancy	VPA dosage (mg/kg)	VPA peak concentration (μg/ml)	Sex of child	Malformation	Number of minor anomalies[a]	Neurological examinations at 6 mos	Neurological examinations at 6 yrs	Neurological examinations at 12–16 yrs	Verbal IQ at 6 yrs	Verbal IQ at 12–16 yrs	EEG at 12–16 yrs	Psychiatric disorder
1	1983	pg	0	30.8	120	m	Spina bifida	23	Died	–	–	93	–	–	–
2	1980	jm	0	30.0	77.0	m	–	5–5	23	–	MND2	–	–	Focal slowing	Anxiety
3	1981	jm	0	27.8	170.0	m	Cranio-stenosis	22–5	17	MND2	MND2	65	–	–	–
4	1983	pg	0	26.5	153	m	Rib hypoplasia	23–11	20	MND1	–	112	–	–	–
5	1982	pg	0	20.7	68	f	–	11	7	–	–	–	–	–	–
6	1983	nc	0	14.1	20.0	f	–	5–5	n	n	n	104	114	n	n
7	1979	pg	0	11.8	16.0	m	–	1	0	n	–	104	–	–	–
8	1977	pg	0	10.9	–	m	–	1–2	23	–	–	–	–	–	–
9	1977	pg	0	10.3	50.0	f	–	4–6	0	n	–	–	–	–	–
10	1983	nc	0	10.0	7.5	m	–	5	0	MND1	n	115	–	–	–
11	1979	pg	1	7.1	–	f	Patent ductus	4–1	0	n	n	98	–	–	–
12	1983	nc	0	4.2	–	m	–	5–0	0	n	MND2	106	89	Focal slowing/photosensitivity	Dyslexia
13	1980	pg	0	–	5.5	f	–	2–0	0	n	n	98	95	n	–
14	1982	jm	2	4.0	42.0	m	–	5–2	0	–	–	Learning retarded	Learning retarded	–	Language
15	1980	pg	2	–	–	F	–	4	5	–	–	–	–	–	–

VPA, valproate; pg, primary generalized; jm, juvenile myoclonic; MND, minor neurological dysfunction; nc, nonclassified; n, normal; – not obtained.
[a] Where two figures are given the first indicates abnormalities at birth and the second indicates abnormalities at last examination.

RESULTS

Of the original sample of 15 newborns with VPA exposure during pregnancy, only nine children could be re-examined at five or six years, and four children were retrieved during adolescence, at 12–16 years of age (Table 1). This attrition rate does not differ from that of the total study sample. Nevertheless, the reasons for discontinuation in the study are of interest. One child died in infancy; two children reside outside Germany; four children and/or their families refused further participation; and three children repeatedly failed to keep appointments. Table 1 provides the clinical data as fully as possible. The children are presented in descending order of prenatal VPA dosage exposure.

Epilepsy in 12 mothers was classified as primary generalized, of whom three have juvenile myoclonic epilepsy. For three mothers classification was not possible due to failure to appear for neurology appointments. Three mothers experienced tonic-clonic seizures during pregnancy. They belonged to the subgroup with a lower dosage of VPA. Peak plasma concentrations above 100 μg/ml during pregnancy were measured in three women, and these women had also received very high mean VPA dosages of 25–31 mg/kg bodyweight. Note that dosage and peak concentration do not correlate completely. The three mothers with very high dosage and very high peak plasma concentrations all gave birth to a malformed child. Child 1 died at seven weeks because of ascending infection of its spina bifida aperta; child 3 was born with a craniostenosis; child 4 was born with hypoplasia of the first ribs and dysplasia of the sternum. Only one child with a malformation, child 11, was born to a mother with low dosage and low plasma concentration. This malformation however, a patent ductus arteriosus, resolved spontaneously within the first year. Children with higher and lower dosage exposure, show various indications of cerebral dysfunction. Child 3, already presented with craniostenosis, exhibited in the follow-up visits a complex neurological and intellectual impairment, psychiatric disorder and EEG abnormalities. Child 12, however, exposed to a low dose of VPA (with unknown peak plasma concentration), had performed normally in the preschool years, but unexpectedly developed abnormal findings during school, such as motor dys-coordination and muscular hypotonia, dyslexia, and focal slowing and photosensitivity in the EEG. Child 13, another low-dose child, received a psychiatric diagnosis of specific language disorder. The learning retardation of child 14 cannot be ascribed to intrauterine drug exposure as he had a bacterial meningitis as a toddler. The family discontinued participation in the study. Of the four children reassessed in early adolescence, only one youngster had normal brain functioning; of the remaining three children, brain disorders were remarkable, and in one case even severe.

DISCUSSION

At the onset of the study, VPA was not known to be teratogenic. There were, however, warnings from animal studies. Nau *et al.* (1981b) had found exencephalies in mouse fetuses. The dosages administered to the mother animals were tenfold higher than those given to humans and half-lives were very short. The rat was therefore considered a very poor animal model for human conditions. Unfortunately, we were to learn otherwise. When a single high dose of VPA is applied, a peak concentration can result in a disproportionately high free fraction because of saturation of the protein binding. In the fetus the free fraction of VPA is much higher than in the newborn and in the mother, exceeding 50% of the total fraction (Nau, 1986; Nau and Krauer, 1986). In animal experiments, high free fractions led to a high percentage of malformed animals (Nau and Krauer, 1986). Investigators from the Berlin study group could demonstrate that a high VPA free fraction alters the proportions of folate metabolites. The formylated tetrahydrofolates, especially folinic acid, decrease; tetrahydrofolate increases (Wegner and Mau, 1992). This alteration may lead to deficiency of the active metabolites because folates are involved in the biochemical reactions of various proteins necessary for cell growth and differentiation in early organogenesis. The embryotoxicity of VPA is seen here. The target tissue for VPA in the fetus is the neuroepithelium. This could be proved by labelling VPA with [14]C (Dencker *et al.*, 1990)

The data of the folate alterations and the accumulation of VPA in the neuroepithelium of the fetus are corroborated by the Vitamin Study Research Group of the Medical Research Council (MRC, 1991). Nonepileptic women who had already delivered a child with spina bifida and were therefore considered at risk of recurrence for neural tube defects in future pregnancies, were included in a randomized double-blind trial. Supplementation with folic acid during pregnancy acted significantly as a protective factor in reducing the recurrence risk.

The joint European prospective study of human teratogenesis associated with maternal epilepsy, in which the Berlin data are included (Samren *et al.*, 1997), presented convincing evidence that children exposed to antiepileptic drugs prenatally bear an altogether 2.3-fold higher risk of major malformations than do controls. In children exposed to VPA as a monotherapy of the mother, the relative risk of major malformations is increased to 4.9. VPA exceeds teratogenicity of other antiepileptic drugs with respect to specificity of malformation, that is, to neural tube defects. In children of mothers treated with a VPA monotherapy the absolute risk of neural tube defect is 3.8%.

This analysis adds another dimension, which is the occurrence of major or minor cerebral dysfunction in later childhood years. Admittedly, the sample is small and the results only descriptive. But to the authors' knowledge no other follow-up of VPA-exposed children exists. Even in this small sample the high number of children with major and minor anomalies, and with major or minor cerebral dysfunctions is appalling. Four children are known to exhibit functional disabilities of the brain. For two children it cannot be proved convincingly that their difficulties result only from VPA teratogenicity, although VPA would be a strong candidate. In one child the brain damage is clearly caused by a bacterial meningitis. In the fifth child, however, brain damage ensued from a malformation of craniostenosis. This major anomaly and additional minor anomalies, typically associated with VPA, strongly suggest a VPA-teratogenesis. Numbers are far too small to draw any conclusions as to whether VPA also produces functional abnormalities besides the now-known teratogenic action to the neuroepithelium. There is a further need to follow-up VPA-exposed children worldwide.

CONCLUSIONS

These data represent a warning that VPA should be used very cautiously with young epileptic women at reproductive age.

1) Women should be treated with the lowest effective dose possible.
2) Doses should be divided into three portions daily, or retard/slow release formulations should be used, to prevent peak concentrations in the fetal tissue.
3) Blood concentrations should always be below 100 μg/ml.
4) A low-dose folic acid (0.4 mg) substitution is recommended before and in the first trimester of pregnancy.
5) Ultrasound sonography in the second trimester should control for neural tube defects and other skeletal defects of the fetus.
6) If a neural tube defect is suspected, alpha-fetoprotein concentration from the blood and amniotic fluid can substantiate the diagnosis.

ACKNOWLEDGEMENTS

This chapter is dedicated to Gertrud Beck-Mannagetta who died in 1996. She participated in the study as a neurologist. Her caring for the epileptic mothers in this study will be remembered as exemplary. We also pay remembrance to her as our dear friend and colleague. We miss her very much. The authors are grateful to Suzanne Spencer, Seattle, Washington, for comments and help with the English.

REFERENCES

Commission on Classification and Terminology of the International League against Epilepsy (1989). Proposal for revised classification of epilepsies and epileptic syndromes. *Epilepsia* **30**, 389–399.

Dencker, L., Nau, H. and D'Argy, R. (1990). Marked accumulation of valproic acid in embryonic neuroepithelium of the mouse during early organogensis. *Teratology* **41**, 699–676.

Eggert, D. (1975). *Hannover-Wechsler Intelligenztest für das Vorschulalter (HAWIVA)*. Huber, Bern.

Jäger-Roman, E., Deichl, A. and Jakob, S. *et al.* (1986). Fetal growth, major malformations, and minor anomalies in infants, born to women receiving valproic acid. *J Pediatrics* **108**, 997–1003.

Lindhout, D. and Meinardi, H. (1984). Spina bifida and *in-vitro* exposure to valproate. *Lancet* **2**, 396.

Lindhout, D., Meinardi, H. and Barth, P.G. (1982). Hazards of fetal exposure to drug combinations. In: Janz, D., Bossi, L., Dam, M., Helge, H., Richens, D. and Schmidt, D. (Eds), *Epilepsy, Pregnancy and the Child*. Raven Press, New York, pp. 275–281.

MRC Vitamin Study Research Group (1991). Prevention of neural tube defects: results of the Medical Research Council Vitamin Group. *Lancet* **338**, 131–137.

Nau, H. (1986). Transfer of valproic acid and its main active unsaturated metabolite to the gestational tissue: correlation with neural tube defect formation in the mouse. *Teratology* **33**, 21–27.

Nau, H., Rating, D., Koch, S., Häuser, I. and Helge, H. (1981a). Valproic acid and its metabolites: placental transfer, neonatal pharmakokinetics, transfer via mother's milk, and clinical status in neonates of epileptic mothers. *J Pharmacol Exp Ther* **219**, 768–777.

Nau, H., Zierer, R., Spielmann, H., Neubert, D. and Gansau, C. (1981b). A new model for embryotoxicity testing: teratogenicity and pharmakokinetics of valproic acid, following constant rate administration in the mouse using human therapeutic drugs and metabolite concentrations. *Life Sci* **29**, 2803–2813.

Nau, H. and Krauer, B. (1986). Serum protein binding of valproic acid in fetus-mother pairs throughout pregnancy: correlation with oxytocin administration and albumin free fatty acid concentrations. *J Clin Pharmacol* **26**, 215–221.

Omzigt, J., Los, F.J., Grobbee, D.E. *et al.* (1992). The risk of spina bifida aperta after first trimester exposure to valproate in a prenatal cohort. *Neurology* **42**, 119–125.

Robert, E. and Gibaud, P. (1982). Maternal valproic acid and congenital neural tube defects. *Lancet* **2**, 934.

Samren, E.B., van Duijn, C.M., Koch, S. *et al.* (1997). Maternal use of antiepileptic drugs and the risk of major malfomations: a joint European prospective study of human teratogenesis associated with maternal epilepsy. *Epilepsia* **38**, 981–990.

Steinhausen, H.-C., Lösche, G., Koch, S. and Helge, H. (1994). The psychological development of children of epileptic parents. Study design and comparative findings. *Acta Paediatr* **42**, 83–88.

Tewes, U. (1983). In: Hg (Ed.) *Hamburg-Wechsler Intelligenztest für Kinder (HAWIK-R)*, revised edition. Huber, Bern.

Tewes, U. (1991). In: Hg (Ed.) *Hamburg-Wechsler Intelligenztest für Erwachsene (HAWIE-E)*. Huber, Bern.

Touwen, B.C.L. (1979). Examination of the child with minor neurological dysfunction. In: *Clinics in Developmental Medicine*. Heinemann Medical, London.

Wegner, C. and Mau, H. (1992). Valproate alters embryonic folate metabolism during organogenesis: implications for the mechanism of teratogenesis of this antiepileptic drug. *Neurology* **42** (suppl 5), 17–24.

World Health Organization (1993). *Diagnostic Criteria for Research*. Huber, Bern.

Juvenile Myoclonic Epilepsy: The Janz Syndrome
Edited by Bettina Schmitz and Thomas Sander
© 2000 Wrightson Biomedical Publishing Ltd

13

Clinical Genetics in Subtypes of Idiopathic Generalized Epilepsies

BETTINA SCHMITZ,[a] ULRIKE SAILER,[b] THOMAS SANDER,[a] GERHARD BAUER[b] and DIETER JANZ[a]

[a]*Department of Neurology, Charité Medical Faculty, Virchow Campus, Humboldt University, Berlin, Germany*
[b]*Department of Neurology, University Hospital, Innsbruck, Austria*

INTRODUCTION

Genetic determinants play a significant role in the manifestation of epileptic seizures. However, only a minority of epilepsies (about 1%) display simple Mendelian modes of inheritance and single gene mutations. For most types of epilepsy modes of inheritance are complex. Furthermore, it is assumed that the epileptic phenotype arises from the interaction of several genes and environmental factors. In complex genetic disorders such as epilepsy there is a lack of a direct correspondence between genotype and phenotype due to heterogeneity and genetic variability. Heterogeneity means that identical or similar phenotypes may be traced down to different genotypes. Genetic variability means that one genotype may be expressed as different phenotypes. To disentangle this complicated genotype–phenotype relationship a close co-operation between clinical epileptologists and molecular geneticists is crucial. Since the efficacy of molecular research depends on the quality of the analysed material, a major task of clinical studies is the identification of suitable, well defined phenotypes.

A number of methodological problems should be considered when looking at clinical genetic research. Penetrance is defined by the proportion of persons with a certain genotype who develop a corresponding phenotype. In epilepsy, particularly in idiopathic syndromes, penetrance is not only incomplete but also strongly age-dependent, with an almost age-specific appearance and disappearance of seizures and/or EEG traits. This phenomenon requires consideration when looking at vertical transmission patterns within families. Figure 1 demonstrates the cumulative incidence of seizure disorders

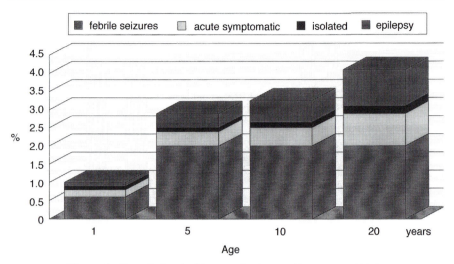

Figure 1. Cumulative incidence of seizures (Annegers, 1991).

to the age of 20, stressing two important methodological issues. First, an age correction is necessary in family studies including young family members who are not yet affected. Secondly, a four-fold difference of seizure occurrence can be obtained simply by using different definitions of an affected relative. Thus, it is important to define seizure disorders clearly. A methodological dilemma arises from the fact that the more representative population-based studies suffer the disadvantage of underreporting of mild symptoms (which is important, particularly for benign syndromes such as pure juvenile myoclonic epilepsy (JME)) and false diagnosis while family studies, which generally provide better clinical data, are sometimes biased by unknown ascertainment procedures which often favour families with multiple affected members who are concordant for a specific epilepsy syndrome.

CLINICAL GENETICS OF EPILEPSY

There are several lines of evidence for a genetic contribution to epilepsy (Table 1). First, we know Mendelian disorders, such as tuberous sclerosis, which are associated with seizures. Secondly, as will be described in detail in the following chapters, for some epilepsy syndromes genes have already been identified. Thirdly, we have animal models which display different monogenic epilepsy syndromes. Fourthly, there is the well-known familial aggregation of epilepsies.

When looking at the offspring risks for epilepsy, there have been consistent estimates of about 3–4% across eight studies which cover the last six

Table 1. Evidence for genetic contribution to epilepsy

1) Genetic animal models
2) Familial aggregation
3) Twin studies
4) Mendelian disorders associated with epilepsy
5) Identified genes in some epilepsies

decades (Table 2). This is clearly increased compared with the risk of developing epilepsy in the general population which is of the order of 1%.

While the increased familial recurrence rate could still be explained by a common environmental factor, twin studies have shown higher concordance rates in monozygotic twins as compared with dizygotic twins. Table 3 summarizes community-based twin studies published between 1965 and 1998. While the risk for a dizygotic twin of developing epilepsy is increased to 5–10%, the risk for monozygotic twins is even higher (approximately four times higher than for dizygotic twins). However, concordance estimates vary widely

Table 2. Offspring risk for epilepsy.

Conrad	1937	4.5%
Alström	1950	3.0%
Harvald	1954	4.4%
Lennox	1951	2.7%
Tsuboi and Endo	1977	2.4%
Annegers *et al.*	1976	3.6%
Beck-Mannagetta *et al.*	1989	4.6%

Table 3. Concordance (%) for epilepsy in twins.

		n	*Monozygotic*	*Dizygotic*
Harvald	1954	127	37	10
Corey *et al.*	1990	280	19	7
Sillanpää *et al.*	1991	188	10	5
Berkovic *et al.*	1998	253	44	10

between studies. This is likely to be related to differences in the diagnosis and definition of seizures which unfortunately have not been clarified in earlier studies.

Which factors increase the risk for epilepsy in children of parents suffering from epilepsy? Figures 2 and 3 summarize results from various epidemiological studies (Anderson *et al.*, 1997). Compared with the 1% risk for epilepsy in

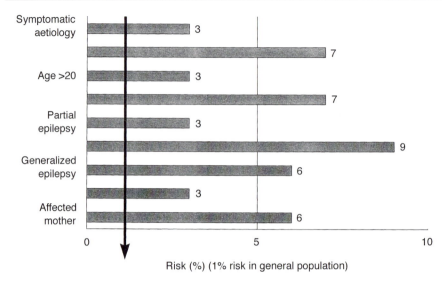

Figure 2. Offspring risk for epilepsy to age 20 (adapted from Anderson et al., 1997).

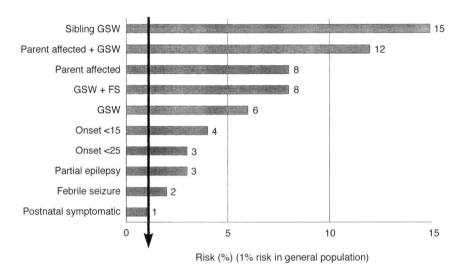

Figure 3. Sibling risk for epilepsy to age 20 (adapted from Anderson et al., 1997).

the general population, the offspring risk rises to 7% when the parent's epilepsy is idiopathic. The risk is also 7% when seizures start early, prior to age 20. The risk is 9% when the parent has absence seizures. Children of mothers with epilepsy have a higher risk of developing epilepsy than children

Table 4. Generalized epilepsies: risk for epilepsy in relatives
(Beck–Mannagetta, 1992).

Proband's syndrome	Sibling risk	Offspring risk
BNS	4%	?
LGS	5%	?
CAE	5–10%	7%
JAE	5%	5%
JME	5–7%	7%
GTCSA	3%	9%

BNS, Blitz-Nick-Salaam seizures (infantile spasms); LGS,
Lennox–Gastaut syndrome; CAE, childhood absence epilepsy; JAE,
juvenile absence epilepsy; JME, juvenile myoclonic epilepsy; GTCSA,
generalized tonic-clonic seizures on awakening.

of fathers with epilepsy – an unexplained observation referred to as maternal
preponderance (Ottmann *et al.*, 1989). The corresponding synopsis of studies
on recurrence risks for siblings of affected probands is given in Figure 3. The
risk is not increased when the proband has a postnatally acquired symptomatic
epilepsy. Age of onset again plays a significant role, with a higher risk associated with an early age of onset. The risk is increased when the proband
displays specific EEG features typical for idiopathic epilepsies: generalized
spikes and waves and photosensitivity. It is further raised when there is an
affected parent in addition to an affected sibling, and the risk is as high as 15%
for a sibling who displays generalized spikes and waves on the EEG.

When looking at specific epilepsy syndromes, community-based studies are
of little value due to their insensitivity. One therefore has to refer to hospi-
tal-based family studies (Beck-Mannagetta and Janz, 1991). Recurrence risks
for siblings of probands suffering from West syndrome and Lennox–Gastaut
syndrome which occur at an early age is 4%. For these severe epileptic
syndromes there are understandably little data on offspring. In one study one
of 7 children from parents with myoclonic-astatic seizures had epilepsy
(Beck-Mannagetta et al. 1994). For the idiopathic generalized syndromes,
recurrence risk for offspring is in the order of 5–7%. This applies to all
idiopathic generalized epilepsy syndromes (Table 4). The figures for siblings
are rather similar, with just minor variations, the only exception being that
the risk for siblings of childhood absence epilepsies (CAE) might be as high
as 10%. There are few data on children of probands with generalized tonic
clonic seizures on awakening (GTCSA). The only existing study suggests an
offspring risk for epilepsy of 9% (Purucker, 1994).

There are few data with respect to focal epilepsies. Recurrence risks in
first-degree relatives of probands suffering from cryptogenic or symptomatic
focal epilepsies seem to be somewhat elevated (in the order of 3%; Beck-
Mannagetta, 1992), suggesting that genetic factors contribute to the manifes-

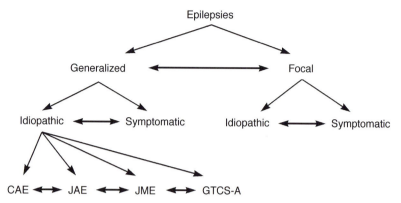

Figure 4. Classification of the epilepsies: CAE, childhood absence epilepsy; JAE, juvenile absence epilepsy; JME, juvenile myoclonic epilepsy; GTCS-A, generalized tonic–clonic seizures on awakening (adapted from Berkovic *et al.*, 1994).

tation of symptomatic epilepsies by lowering the seizure threshold. Recurrence risks for siblings of probands with benign idiopathic focal epilepsies have been found to be as high as 15% (Heijbel *et al.*, 1975). There are no data on offspring risks for this type of epilepsy although these must be expected to be increased.

CLINICAL GENETICS OF IDIOPATHIC GENERALIZED EPILEPSY (IGE) SUBTYPES: 'LUMPING OR SPLITTING?'

The simplification of the International Classification of Epilepsies (Figure 4) emphasizes the major IGE subtypes (Berkovic *et al.*, 1994). The double-headed arrows indicate overlap between categories which is of particular importance for the four syndromes of CAE, juvenile absence epilepsy (JAE), JME and GTCSA. What do these IGE subtypes have in common, justifying lumping them together, and what are the differences, justifying splitting them up?

The first line of evidence that the common IGE subtypes form a biological continuum comes from clinical studies stressing the intraindividual syndromic overlap. The graph from Janz's textbook on epilepsies from 1998 (Figure 5) demonstrates the ages of onset of generalized epilepsies which have peaks ranging from early childhood to adolescence (Janz, 1998). In a more recent case series by Janz the ages of onset for the common IGE subtypes were given as follows: in CAE 5–10 years, in JAE 10–15 years, and in JME 12–18 years (Janz, 1990). Thus, ages of onset seem to be restricted to a limited lifespan in these common petit mal syndromes. Manifestation ages of GTCSA stretch, however, from six to 22 years.

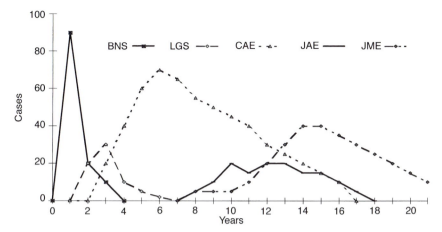

Figure 5. Age of onset in generalized epilepsy subtypes (Janz, 1998). BNS, Blitz–Nick–Salaam seizures (infantile spasms); LGS, Lennox–Gastaut syndrome; CAE, childhood absence epilepsy; JAE, juvenile absence epilepsy; JME, juvenile myoclonic epilepsy.

Differentiation of the two absence epilepsy syndromes is often not possible. The definition of the syndromes is to a certain degree artificial and therefore controversial (Berkovic *et al.*, 1987). The absence syndromes are defined by seizure frequency and age of onset. When using seizure frequency as the major diagnostic criterion (Figure 6) (one or more absences daily in CAE, less than one seizure daily in JAE) it becomes obvious that the ages of onset

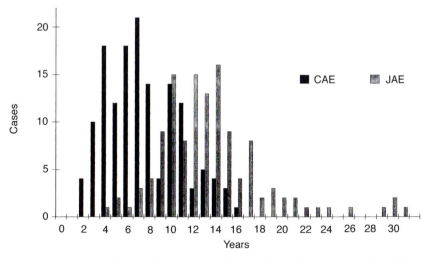

Figure 6. Age of onset in absence epilepsies ($n = 142$) (Janz *et al.*, 1994).

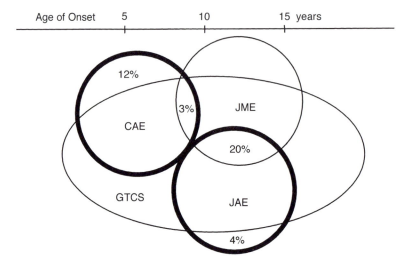

Figure 7. Incidence of myoclonic seizures in absence epilepsies (*n* = 306) (Janz, 1990). CAE, childhood absence epilepsy; JME, juvenile myoclonic epilepsy; GTCS, generalized tonic–clonic seizures; JAE, juvenile absence epilepsy.

are not distinct, but if superimposed rather form a continuous curve (Janz *et al.*, 1994).

Figures 7 and 8 emphasize the intraindividual syndromic overlap between absence epilepsies and JME (Janz, 1990). In this series only 3% of probands diagnosed with CAE developed JME, but 20% of JAE probands developed JME in their later course.

Figure 8 highlights the syndromic overlap between probands diagnosed as JME and the two absence syndromes. Again, there was a higher overlap between JME and JAE as compared with JME and CAE, being 22% and 6% respectively. These data suggest a closer link between JME and JAE than between JME and CAE. This finding, however, might be an artefact related to the different ages of onset which are closer between JME and JAE than between JME and CAE. There is evidence for a selection bias since there are studies in the literature suggesting a higher rate of JME in probands with CAE. Wirrell *et al.* (1996) found a proportion of 15% of 81 CAE probands (defined by the occurrence of pyknoleptic absences prior to puberty) who had developed JME at follow-up. This series is also characterized by a low remission rate of 65% which suggests that effective treatment prevents progression into JME.

Combinations with GTCS, particularly with GTCSA, are very common in all three petit mal subtypes, occurring in 88% of CAE probands, 96% of JAE probands and 93% of JME probands with GM seizures (Janz, 1989).

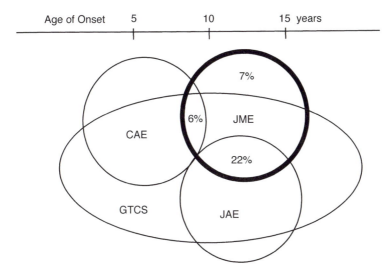

Figure 8. Incidence of absences in JME (*n* = 186) (Janz, 1990). CAE, childhood absence epilepsy; JME, juvenile myoclonic epilepsy; GTCS, generalized tonic–clonic seizures; JAE, juvenile absence epilepsy.

These data may be biased because they refer to a hospital series, where underdiagnosis of pure petit mal epilepsies can be assumed.

The other indicator for a close link between the common IGE subtypes is based on data from family studies looking at the rate of intrafamilial syndromic concordance. The data from an Australian twin study suggest that with respect to major syndromic categories there is a higher concordance rate in monozygotic twins as compared with dizygotic twins for generalized epilepsies and idiopathic focal epilepsies (Berkovic *et al.*, 1998). The concordance rate for IGEs was 0.76 in monozygotic twins and 0.26 in dizygotic twins. For idiopathic focal epilepsies concordance rates were 0.36 and 0.05 for monozygotic and dizygotic twins respectively. The syndromic concordance rate for cryptogenic focal epilepsies, however, was identical when comparing monozygotic and dizygotic twins (0.33). The authors conclude that there are syndrome-specific genes that determine human epilepsy. However, their syndromic classification (idiopathic and symptomatic generalized, idiopathic, cryptogenic and symptomatic focal) is rather gross and does not distinguish IGE subtypes.

Since prognosis of epilepsies is very variable, it is important, for the purposes of genetic research as well as for genetic counselling, to know which types of epilepsy occur in affected relatives. The data from an earlier Berlin pedigree study are summarized in Figure 9, demonstrating epileptic syndromes seen in relatives of probands suffering from generalized epilepsies (Beck-Mannagetta and Janz, 1991). There was only one relative who had

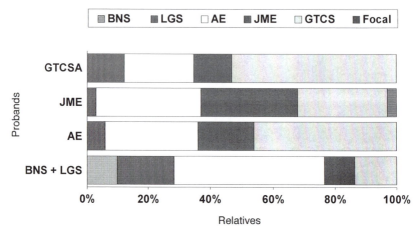

Figure 9. Syndromes in first-degree relatives of probands with IGE ($n = 91$) (Beck-Mannagetta and Janz, 1991). BNS, Blitz–Nick–Salaam seizures (infantile spasms); LGS, Lennox–Gastaut syndrome; AE, absence epilepsy; JME, juvenile myoclonic epilepsy; GTCSA, generalized tonic–clonic seizures on awakening.

a focal epilepsy; all others were classified as having a generalized epilepsy syndrome. The risk for focal epilepsies in relatives of generalized epilepsies can therefore be ignored. The only case of West syndrome was seen in a relative of a proband who had the syndrome himself. Among the idiopathic IGE subtypes there was a considerable intrafamilial syndromic overlap leading to the question of their genetic relationship.

The authors have recently analysed the clinical data from 118 multiplex families ascertained through a proband with a definite diagnosis of either CAE, JAE or JME and a first-degree relative with at least one unprovoked generalized seizure (Schmitz et al., 1995) (Table 5). Absence epilepsies were classified according to seizure frequency. The study was based on a series of multiplex epilepsy families which were collected over many years by two epilepsy centres (Berlin, Germany and Innsbruck, Austria) in collaboration with a number of international epileptologists. The objective of the clinical analysis was to extract as much information as possible in order to identify familial patterns which may suggest specific modes of inheritance in order to further focus and guide our molecular genetic studies. The aim was to identify families which from a clinical point of view seem to share common genetic backgrounds.

Within the 118 included families there were 155 affected relatives, between one and four per family (mean 2.3). These were 22 affected mothers (19%), 27 fathers (23%), 48 affected sisters out of a total of 173 sisters (28%), 41 of 164 brothers (25%), six of 52 daughters (12%) and eleven of 56 sons (20%).

Table 5. Clinical and EEG data of probands with CAE, JAE or JME (n = 118[a]).

	CAE n = 33	*JAE* n = 39	*JME* n = 54
Mean age of onset (range)	6.4 years (2–12)	14.1 years (8–26)	15.3 years (9–27)
Mean age at investigation (range)	28.0 years (8–49)	35.3 years (16–77)	29.6 years (13–60)
Mean family size (range)	6.9 (4–18)	7.5 (4–16)	6.2 (3–14)
Mean affected relatives (range)	1.3 (1–4)	1.26 (1–4)	1.35 (1–4)
Females/males	19/14	23/16	37/17
Additional petit mal	1 JME	7 JME	8 AE
Febrile convulsions	1	2	2
No GTCS	7	3	8
Single GTCS	1	1	6
Two to six GTCS	12	2	10
More than six GTCS	13	26	24
GTCS on awakening	17	24	31
GTCS resting	3	2	2
GTCS sleep	5	1	1
GTCS random	1	5	2
Patients with EEG	33	39	52
3/s spike-waves[b]	24	23	13
Slow spike-waves	1	0	0
Irregular spike-waves	1	3	6
Polyspike-waves	8	6	18
Polyspikes	5	1	3
Spikes	2	15	6
Sharp slow-waves	1	3	2
Sharp waves	3	17	4
Paroxysmal slow	1	4	1
No generalized epileptiform activity	2	0	8
Abnormal background activity	8	3	3
Focal slowing	1	2	2
Focal specific	1	2	1
Photosensitivity	7	9	16

[a]Eight cases with combinations of AE and JME were considered twice.
[b]3/s or faster spike-waves.
CAE, childhood absence epilepsy; JAE, juvenile absence epilepsy; JME, juvenile myoclonic epilepsy; AE, absence epilepsy; GTCS, generalized tonic-clonic seizures.

Figure 10 demonstrates the syndromic concordance between probands and affected relatives in 165 kin-pairs. (The number of kin-pairs exceeds the number of affected relatives by *n* = 10 because eight probands with a combination of absence epilepsies with JME were considered twice. One of these had three affected relatives, resulting in three extra kin-pairs.) Among relatives, CAE, JAE and JME syndromes showed a semispecific distribution according to the proband's syndrome. There were comparable syndromic concordance rates of 41%, 41% and 45% for CAE, JAE and JME, respectively. JAE occurred in 19% of relatives of probands with CAE; the same proportion of 19% JAE was seen in relatives of JME probands. Only 2% of relatives of CAE probands displayed JME and only 8% of relatives of JME

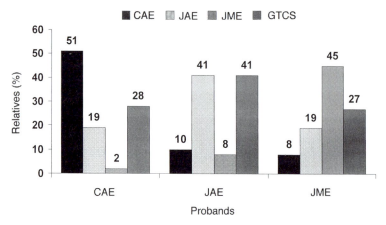

Figure 10. Syndrome concordance in 165 kin-pairs. CAE, childhood absence epilepsy; JAE, juvenile absence epilepsy; JME, juvenile myoclonic epilepsy; GTCS, generalized tonic–clonic seizures.

probands displayed CAE. Pure GTCS occurred in 27% and 28% of relatives of CAE and JME respectively, but in 41% of relatives of JAE probands.

DISCUSSION

These families are likely to be biased towards concordant syndromes. Therefore the intrafamilial combination of different IGE subtypes is the more significant finding, suggesting that these syndromes share a common genetic background.

In order to identify factors associated with syndromic concordance the authors compared probands with concordant relatives to probands with discordant relatives. For JME probands there were neither clinical nor EEG parameters associated with syndromic concordance. For probands with CAE, mean age of onset was significantly lower in concordant probands as compared with nonconcordant probands. The authors then looked at patients with early onset of CAE (six years or younger) and compared them to CAE probands with a later manifestation age. It is interesting to note that there was a preponderance of CAE in relatives of probands with early-onset CAE and a tendency towards JAE in relatives of probands with late-onset CAE. It is also worth noting that in the subgroup of CAE there was a significant correlation of manifestation ages of petit mal seizures between probands and affected relatives (Pearson's correlation coefficient = 0.52, $p < 0.001$). These data suggest that the susceptibility to developing seizures at a certain age might be inherited.

These results with respect to intrafamilial phenotype concordance confirm the semi-specific overlap between the three petit mal syndromes CAE, JAE and JME which has been described in the literature by the authors' group and other investigators (Beck-Mannagetta and Janz, 1991; Delgado-Escueta *et al.*, 1990). In the Italian sample of multiplex families there was a lower intrafamilial association between CAE and JME (Italian League Against Epilepsy Genetic Collaborative Group, 1993). This series is, however, unusual because of the relatively low number of JME families ($n = 7$) as compared with CAE ($n = 28$) and the complete lack of JAE families.

In the authors' material, there is a relatively high concordance rate within families both of CAE and JME probands, and a lower concordance rate in families of JAE probands. There is little intrafamilial overlap between CAE and JME, but there is a relatively high proportion of JAE relatives in both families of CAE probands and families of JME probands. In JAE families there was the highest proportion of pure GTCS epilepsies among affected relatives, which demonstrates the known syndromic link between JAE and GTCS (Commission on Classification and Terminology of the ILAE, 1989). It is also possible that infrequent absences were missed in some of these relatives with GTCS, thus leading to an underestimation of concordance for JAE.

In order to avoid unclassifiable cases, absence epilepsies were defined exclusively according to seizure frequency and age of onset was ignored. Part of the intrafamilial overlap between CAE and JAE is a consequence of this artificial definition, since late-onset CAE in probands was relatively often associated with JAE in relatives. Seven of the eight probands with petit mal combinations were between JAE and JME. These findings support the view that JAE holds an intermediate position with soft borders to both CAE and JME.

CONCLUSION

There is strong and accumulating evidence for genetic contributions to epilepsy in general, and in particular to the idiopathic generalized syndromes. The recurrence risks for epilepsy in the offspring of patients exhibiting the common IGEs is in the order of 5–7%, and – important for genetic counselling – affected relatives are likely to have one of the IGE syndromes, which in general are benign disorders with a relatively mild impact on quality of life.

The sporadic appearance of most cases of epilepsy, the relatively low increase of epilepsy in relatives of affected individuals, and the range of clinical types of epilepsy within families do not suggest that a major gene with high penetrance will be found for all types of epilepsy or even for the more common clinical subgroups. It is more likely that there are several suscepti-bility alleles which increase the risk for all types of seizure although they may enhance the risk for some types of seizure more than others (Annegers, 1991). The search for such susceptibility alleles has resulted in some promising, some contradictory, and many negative results.

With respect to IGE, recent findings suggest heterogeneity. The EJM1 locus has been shown to be linked with many (Greenberg *et al.*, 1988; Weissbecker *et al.*, 1991; Durner *et al.*, 1992), but not with all JME families (Whitehouse *et al.*, 1993). Linkage could be demonstrated with absences in JME families and with GTCSA but not with random GTCS (Greenberg *et al.*, 1995), and not with absence seizures in families without JME members (Sander *et al.*, 1995).

These results show that even with the rapidly expanding use of molecular studies, family studies remain important. In most molecular studies different epileptic syndromes are 'lumped' together. This approach may be justified by the observed intrafamilial syndromic overlap, but often there is simply no alternative due to the relative rarity of multiplex families and the lack of detailed clinical information on relatives.

The intraindividual and intrafamilial overlap within the generalized epilepsy syndromes suggests a biological continuum and a shared genetic background. A better selection of families may help to reduce false-negative and contradictory findings. In order to further define the genetics of JME and its IGE siblings future family studies should consider more specific clinical data beyond age of onset, seizure types and classical EEG patterns. With respect to JME these data should include factors which it has been only recently learned are associated with Janz syndrome, such as specific modes of seizure precipitation, sophisticated electrophysiological findings and neuropsychological profiles, as well as results from functional and structural imaging studies.

REFERENCES

Alström, C.G. (1950). A study of epilepsy in its clinical, social and genetic aspects. *Acta Psychiatr Kbh* **63**, 1–284.

Anderson, V.E., Andermann, E. and Hauser, W.A. (1997). Genetic counseling. In: Engel, J. and Pedley, T.A. (Eds), *Epilepsy: A Comprehensive Textbook*. Lippincott Raven, Philadelphia, PA, pp. 225–230.

Annegers, J.F. (1991). The use of analytic epidemiologic methods in family studies of epilepsy. *Epilepsy Res* (suppl 4), 139–146.

Annegers, J.F., Hauser, W.A., Elveback, L.R., Anderson, V.E. and Kurland, L.T. (1976). Seizure disorders in offspring of parents with a history of seizures - a maternal-paternal difference? *Epilepsia* **17**, 1–9.

Beck-Mannagetta, G. (1992). Genetik und Genetische Beratung. In: Hopf, H.C., Poeck, K. and Schliack, H. (Eds), *Neurologie in Praxis und Klinik*. Thieme, Stuttgart, pp. 3.57–3.63.

Beck-Mannagetta, G. and Janz, D. (1991). Syndrome related genetics in generalized epilepsy. *Epilepsy Res* **32** (suppl), 105–111.

Beck-Mannagetta, G., Janz, D., Hoffmeister, U., Behl, I. and Scholz, G. (1989). Morbidity risk for seizures and epilepsy in offspring of patients with epilepsy. In: Beck-Mannagetta, G., Anderson, V.E., Doose, H., Janz, D. (Eds), *Genetics of the Epilepsies*, Springer, Berlin, pp. 119–26.

Beck-Mannagetta, G., Dehe-Steffens, C., Schmitz, B. and Janz, D. (1994). Genetic aspects of epilepsies with myoclonic-astatic seizures. In: Wolf, P. (Ed.), *Epileptic Seizures and Syndromes*, John Libbey, London, pp. 165–168.

Berkovic, S.F, Andermann, F., Andermann, E. and Gloor, P. (1987). Concepts of absence epilepsies: discrete syndromes or biological continuum? *Neurology* **37**, 993–1000.

Berkovic, S.F., Reutens, D.C., Andermann, E. and Andermann, F. (1994). The epilepsies: specific syndromes or neurobiological continuum? In: Wolf, P. (Ed.), *Epileptic Seizures and Syndromes*. John Libbey, London, pp. 25–40.

Berkovic, S.F., Howell, R.A., Hay, D.A. and Hopper, J.L. (1998). Epilepsies in twins: genetics of the major epilepsy syndromes. *Ann Neurol* **43**, 435–445.

Commission on Classification and Terminology of the International League Against Epilepsy (1989). Proposal for revised classification of epilepsies and epileptic syndromes. *Epilepsia* **30**, 389–399.

Conrad, K. (1937). Erbanlage und Epilepsie. Untersuchung an einer Serie von 253 Zwillingspaaren. *Z Neurol Psychiatr* **153**, 271–326.

Corey, L., Berg, K., Pellock, J., Nance, W. and DeLorenzo, R. (1990). Seizure syndromes in Virginia and Norwegian twin kindreds. *Epilepsia* **31**, 814.

Delgado-Escueta, A.V., Greenberg, D.A., Weissbecker, K.A. *et al.* (1989). Mapping the gene for juvenile myoclonic epilepsy. *Epilepsia* **30** (suppl. 4), 8–18.

Delgado-Escueta, A.V., Greenberg, D., Weissbecker, K. *et al.* (1990). Gene mapping in the idiopathic generalized epilepsies: Juvenile myoclonic epilepsy, childhood absence epilepsy, epilepsy with grand mal on awakening and early childhood myoclonic epilepsy. *Epilepsia* **31** (suppl 3), 19–29.

Durner, M., Janz, D., Zingsem, J. and Greenberg, D.A. (1992). Possible association of juvenile myoclonic epilepsy with HLA-DRw6. *Epilepsia* **33**, 814–816.

Greenberg, D.A., Delgado-Escueta, A.V., Widelitz, H. *et al.* (1988). Juvenile Myoclonic Epilepsy (JME) may be linked to the Bf and HLA region on chromosome 6. *Am J Med Genet* **31**, 185–192.

Greenberg, D.A., Durner, M, Resor, S., Rosenbaum, D. and Shinnar, S. (1995). The genetics of idiopathic generalized epilepsies of adolescent onset: differences between juvenile myoclonic epilepsy and epilepsy with random grand mal and with awakening grand mal. *Neurology* **45**, 942–946.

Harvald, B. (1954). *Heredity in Epilepsy. An Electroencephalographic Study of Relatives of Epileptics*. Ejnar Munksgaard, Copenhagen.

Heijbel, J., Blom, S. and Rasmuson M. (1975) Benign epilepsy of childhood with centro-temporal EEG foci: a genetic study. *Epilepsia* **16**, 285–293.

Italian League Against Epilepsy Genetic Collaborative Group (1993). Concordance of clinical forms of epilepsy in families with several affected members. *Epilepsia* **34**, 819–826.

Janz, D. (1989). Juvenile myoclonic epilepsy: epilepsy with impulsive petit mal. *Cleveland Clin J Medicine* **56** (suppl 1), 23–33.

Janz, D. (1990). Juvenile myoclonic epilepsy. In: Dam, M. and Gram, L. (Eds), *Comprehensive Epileptology*. Raven Press, New York, pp. 171–185.

Janz, D. (1998). *Die Epilepsien, Spezielle Pathologie und Therapie*, second edition. Thieme, Stuttgart (first published 1969).

Janz, D., Beck-Mannagetta, G., Spröder, B., Spröder, J. and Waltz, S. (1994).

Childhood absence epilepsy (pyknolepsy) and juvenile absence epilepsy: one or two syndromes? In: Wolf, P. (Ed.), *Epileptic Seizures and Syndromes.* John Libbey, London, pp. 213–220.

Lennox, W.G. (1951). The heredity of epilepsy as told by relatives and twins. *JAMA* **146**, 529.

Ottmann, R., Annegers, J.F., Hauser, A. and Kurland, L.T. (1989). Higher risk of seizures in offspring of mothers than of fathers with epilepsy. *Epilepsia* **43**, 257–264.

Purucker, H. (1994). *Klinik und klinische Genetik der Epilepsie mit reinen Aufwach-Grand mal.* Thesis, Free University, Berlin.

Sander, T., Hildmann, T., Janz, D. *et al.* (1995) The phenotypic spectrum related to the human epilepsy susceptibility gene 'EJM1'. *Ann Neurol* **38**, 210–217.

Schmitz, B., Sailer, U., Sander, T., Beck-Mannagetta, G., Bauer, G. and Janz, D. (1995). Syndrome related genetics in idiopathic generalized epilepsies. *Epilepsia* **36** (suppl 3), 27.

Sillanpää, M., Koskenvuo, M., Romanov, H. and Kaprio, J. (1991). Genetic factors in epileptic seizures: evidence from a large twin population. *Acta Neurol Scand* **84**, 523–526.

Tsuboi, T. and Endo, S. (1977). Incidence of seizures and EEG abnormalities among offspring of epileptic patients. *Hum Genet* **36**, 173–189.

Weissbecker, K.A., Durner, M., Janz, D., Scaramelli, A., Sparkes, R.S. and Spence, M.A. (1991). Confirmation of linkage between juvenile myoclonic epilepsy and the HLA region on chromosome 6p in families ascertained through juvenile myoclonic epilepsy patients. *Neurology* **41**, 1651–1655.

Whitehouse, W.P., Rees, M., Curtis, D. *et al.* (1993). Linkage analysis of idiopathic generalized epilepsy (IGE) and marker loci on chromosome 6p in families of patients with juvenile myoclonic epilepsy: no evidence for an epilepsy locus in the HLA region. *Am J Hum Genet* **53**, 652–662.

Wirrell, E.C., Camfield, C.S., Camfield, P.R., Gordon, K.E. and Dooley, J.M. (1996). Long-term prognosis of typical childhood absence epilepsy: remission or progression to juvenile myoclonic epilepsy. *Neurology* **47**, 912–918.

14

The Search for Epilepsy Genes in Juvenile Myoclonic Epilepsy: Discoveries Along the Way

ANTONIO V. DELGADO-ESCUETA,[a,b] MARIA E. ALONSO,[c] MARCO T. MEDINA,[a,d] MANYEE N. GEE[a] and G.C.Y. FONG[a]

[a]*California Comprehensive Epilepsy Program, UCLA School of Medicine and West Los Angeles DVA Medical Center*
[b]*UCLA Brain Research Institute, Los Angeles, California, USA*
[c]*National Institute of Neurology and Neurosurgery, Mexico City, Mexico*
[d]*National University of Honduras, Tegucigalpa, Honduras*

INTRODUCTION

In 1955, Janz and Matthes and in 1957, Janz and Christian recognized an epilepsy syndrome in 47 patients called 'impulsive petit mal' characterized by adolescent-onset myoclonic jerks of shoulders and arms which occur usually after awakening. Most patients also had generalized tonic-clonic seizures and some had absences. Sleep deprivation, alcohol intake and fatigue commonly precipitated seizures. In 1958, Castells and Mendilaharsu, at the Montevideo School of Medicine, reported a syndrome similar to impulsive petit mal in 70 patients with 'bilateral and conscious myoclonic epilepsy'. Because these papers from Germany and Uruguay were published in German and Spanish, they were ignored by the neurological and epilepsy literature in the English-speaking world.

Between 1969 and 1975, Delgado-Escueta and Enrile-Bacsal recorded closed-circuit television-electroencephalogram (CCTV-EEG) manifestations of myoclonias and tonic-clonic grand mal seizures in a familial adolescent-onset epilepsy syndrome which was named 'benign myoclonic and tonic-clonic seizures in adolescence and late childhood'. These CCTV-EEG

The authors are members of the Genetic Epilepsy Studies (GENES) International Consortium.

recordings were used during the 1970s for several of the electroencephalography courses at the American Academy of Neurology and were presented in 1980 for genetic linkage studies at a workshop on the genetic basis of the epilepsies held in Minneapolis, Minnesota, USA. During this meeting, the researchers were convinced by Janz that this familial syndrome of adolescence and impulsive petit mal were the same disease. In appreciation of Janz's earlier work, they called the syndrome juvenile myoclonic epilepsy of Janz, or JME (Delgado-Escueta and Enrile-Bacsal, 1984).

Between 1986 and 1988, the authors' laboratory reported that the classic JME locus may be in chromosome 6p, probably outside the HLA region (Greenberg et al., 1987, 1988). In 1995 and 1996, they presented evidence in two large JME families that a JME locus was in chromosome 6p11, some 20 cM below HLA (Serratosa et al., 1996; Liu et al., 1995, 1996). Since then, the authors have mapped three loci for common idiopathic generalized epilepsies, two of which could easily be placed within the JME syndrome. They are (1) childhood absence epilepsy (CAE) that evolves to JME in chromosome 1p (Westling et al., 1996; Westling, 1997); (2) photogenic childhood absence with eyelid myoclonia evolving to JME (Delgado-Escueta et al., 1999); and (3) classic CAE with or without grand mal in chromosome 8q24 (Fong et al., 1998) (see Table 1). They also mapped a locus in chromosome 6q24 for Lafora's disease (Serratosa et al., 1996) and helped identify its mutation (Minassian et al., 1998; Serratosa et al., 1999). This chapter chronicles the quest for epilepsy genes in JME, the discoveries made along the way, and why the authors believe there is more than one 'Janz epilepsy gene'.

LAFORA'S PROGRESSIVE MYOCLONUS EPILEPSY IN 6q24 IS CAUSED BY A MUTATION IN TYROSINE PHOSPHATASE GENE

An autosomal recessive fatal generalized storage disorder, Lafora's disease (LD) initially manifests as myoclonic, tonic-clonic absences, or visual seizures followed by stimuli-sensitive asymmetric myoclonic jerks (Lafora, 1911; Lafora and Glueck, 1911). The average age of onset is 14 years. As the disease progresses, the myoclonus increases in frequency and becomes constant. A rapidly progressive dementia with apraxia and visual loss ensues; patients finally become totally disabled and die after a vegetative period, usually within less than 10 years from first symptoms. The diagnostic procedure of choice is now an armpit skin biopsy where the characteristic periodic acid-Schiff (PAS)-positive cytoplasmic inclusion bodies can be seen in myoepithelial cells of secretory acini of apocrine glands and in cells of the eccrine duct (Carpenter and Karpati, 1981; Busard et al., 1987).

Among 54 LD patients studied in the authors' laboratories, 24 were mistakenly diagnosed in the early part of their illness as having JME.

Table 1. Chromosomal loci of juvenile myoclonic epilepsy (JME) and related idiopathic generalized epilepsies (IGEs).

Syndromes	Clinical characteristics	Chromosome locus
Reported by Delgado-Escueta and co-workers		
1) Classic JME	Adolescent-onset myoclonias simultaneously presenting with or followed within 1–10 years by grand mal tonic-clonic seizures; rare random spanioleptic absences may be present; asymptomatics with diffuse fast multispike wave complexes.	6p11 (Liu et al., 1995; Serratosa et al., 1996)
2) Childhood absence epilepsy (CAE) that evolves to JME	Childhood or adolescent onset as pyknoleptic absences (1–200/day) followed by myoclonic and tonic-clonic seizures during adolescence; asymptomatics with classic 3 Hz spike-waves.	1p (Westling et al., 1996, 1997)
3) Photogenic absence epilepsies with eyelid myoclonia evolving to JME	Childhood or adolescent visual stimuli-induced absences with eyelid myoclonia, grand mal and myoclonias; usually female preponderance.	(to be published)
4) Classic or typical child-hood absence or CAE	Early or mid-childhood onset as pyknoleptic absences (1–200/day) persisting or remitting, with or without grand mal.	8q24 (Gee et al., 1997; Fong et al., 1998)
Reported by Gardiner and co-workers		
5) JME	JME and JME mixed with absences.	15q (Elmslie et al., 1996, 1997)
Reported by Greenberg and co-workers		
6) Pure awakening grand mal syndrome	Clinical phenotype of awakening grand mal.	6p (HLA region) (Greenberg et al., 1996)
7) JME	JME in 2/3 and JME mixed with absences in 1/3 of cases.	6p (HLA region) (Greenberg et al., 1996)
Chromosomal loci reported by Pandolfo and co-workers		
8) IGEs including JME	Mixture of JME, febrile convulsions, grand mal only and absences plus asymptomatics with spike-wave complexes.	8q24 (Zara et al., 1995)
9) IGEs	Mainly asymptomatics with spike-wave EEG phenotype of IGEs and two clinically affected.	3p (Zara et al., 1997)

Because of its rapidly progressive and fatal nature, and because of the continuing appeal of parents for their dying children, the authors made the solution
of Lafora's disease one of their top priorities. Although rare in the USA and
Canada, LD is relatively common in Southern Europe (Italy, France, Spain),
northern Africa, the Middle East, the Karnataka state in southern India, and
parts of the world where a high rate of consanguinity occurs among the
population.

Between 1993 to 1997, several key developments led to the definition of
the LD gene mutation. While screening the genome for linkage to LD,
extended areas of homozygosities were encountered in chromosome 6q23-25
in 18 patients belonging to 10 families, six of which were consanguineous
marriages (families LD1, LD4, LD5, LD9, LD15, LD16, LD17, LD20, LD22,
LD33). Two large inbred families, one from Palestine, Israel, (LD9) and one
from Kentucky, USA, (LD33) each independently proved linkage to chromosome 6q23-25 markers. Thus, in 1995, Serratosa et al. initially mapped the
LD gene to a 17 cM interval in chromosome 6q23-25 and, in 1997, Sainz et
al. reduced the size of the critical LD region to a 2.7 cM interval between
D6S1003 and D6S311. In order to avoid the huge task of identifying and
studying all transcripts in the large 2.7 cM genomic region, the localization
of the LD candidate region was refined by examining for heterozygosities
within the regions of homozygosities in 31 LD patients whose families
showed high posterior probability of linkage ($W_i>0.75$). Analyses which
included homozygosities in eight new informative families from Italy and
Argentina identified informative heterozygosities in six families that significantly reduced the LD candidate region from 2.7 cM to approximately
300 kb, in the vicinity of D6S1703 (Delgado-Escueta et al., 1999). This paved
the way for positional cloning and mutation analyses.

Refined mapping to D6S1703 was further reinforced when Minassian et al.
(1998) detected one family from Brazil with a homozygous microdeletion at
D6S1703. This microdeletion covered approximately 500 kb of DNA at
D6S1703. The genomic DNA sequence of three PAC clones that encom-
passed this microdeletion showed by DNA sequence analyses that only one
gene was present. This novel gene encoded a protein with consensus amino
acid sequence indicative of a tyrosine phosphatase. Using the available
genomic structure of the LD1 gene, Minassian et al. (1998) screened for
mutations in LD patients and found six distinct DNA sequence variations in
tyrosine phosphatase in nine families so far. Six families from Spain showed
a homozygous nonsense mutation that results from a C to T change, leading
to a premature stop codon. One family from the Karnataka region of India
had a homozygous G to T nonsense mutation resulting in a frame stop codon
and a predicted premature termination of the putative LD1 protein. In one
family, from the Appalachian mountains of Kentucky, USA, a homozygous
A to T transition results in a glutamine to leucine change in a residue located

just after the tyrosine phosphatase domain. A homozygous insertion of an A resulting in a frameshift interruption of the tyrosine phosphatase domain was identified in one family from Brazil. The authors' laboratories are now continuing mutation analyses in new families with LD from the middle East, Mexico, Central America and Italy. Serratosa *et al.* (1999), working independently, recently observed mutations in the same novel gene for tyrosine phosphatase in families from Spain, Turkey and Europe.

The authors' laboratories also examined for heterogeneity through the admixture text (H_2 versus H_1) in 22 families with LD and observed significance ($p = 0.0009$ for D6S311 and $p = 0.004$ for D6S310). The estimated proportion of linked families, α, was 75% for D6S311 and 85% for D6S471 (95% confidence interval 0.05–0.99). Extremely low posterior probabilities of linkage ($W_i = 0.002$ to 0.0000) identified four families unlikely to be linked to D6S311. Exclusionary LOD scores and haplotypes in these four families further supported locus heterogeneity in LD. Three families are from Quebec, Canada, and one is from Saudi Arabia. These families form the basis for the search for a second LD gene (Minassian *et al.*, 1999).

THE SYNDROME OF JUVENILE MYOCLONIC EPILEPSY OF JANZ HAS LOCUS HETEROGENEITY (SEE TABLE 1)

Among the 20 to 50 million people with generalized epilepsies, the most common are JME, childhood absence epilepsy (CAE) and pure grand mal on awakening (Hauser and Hesdorffer, 1990; Commission on Classification and Terminology of the ILAE, 1981, 1989). JME is probably the most common form of generalized epilepsy, accounting for 10–30% of all epilepsies (Janz, 1969, 1985). CAE with or without grand mal accounts for another 5–15% of all epilepsies. Grand mal on awakening is reported to account for 22–37% of all epilepsies. However, the authors believe they are less common because CCTV-EEG telemetry or polygraphy show that grand mal seizures are most often preceded by myoclonic seizures or absences (Lee *et al.*, 1987; Loiseau, 1964; Roger *et al.*, 1992).

The authors' GENES international consortium observed four subsyndromes within 144 JME families. The first subsyndrome is classic JME without pyknoleptic absences. Characteristically, myoclonias start in the morning during adolescence, most commonly at 13–15 years of age. Diffuse high-amplitude EEG polyspikes accompany clinical myoclonias and are usually triggered by sleep deprivation, alcohol and fatigue. Two years after the onset of adolescent awakening myoclonias, grand mal convulsions appear. Rare spanioleptic absences may appear during adolescence but are difficult to capture on CCTV-EEG telemetry. Female sex preponderance is present (three to two ratio) and photosensitivity is rare. Twenty-eight per cent of families are multiplex or multigenerational. Affected family members have grand mal or JME. Absences are rare in affected members, e.g. one in 21 affected members. The segregation ratio across matings is 0.14 and across normal by affected matings is 0.54. Classic JME accounted for 45% of all JME in the authors' dataset.

The second subsyndrome of JME starts during late childhood as pyknoleptic absences with 3 Hz spike and wave complexes as well as 4–6 Hz spike- or polyspike-wave complexes. During adolescence, myoclonias and grand mal convulsions follow. This subsyndrome accounted for 27% of all JME cases in the authors' dataset.

The third subsyndrome of JME starts with pyknoleptic absences, myoclonias and grand mal convulsions all at the same time during adolescence. EEGs show interictal 4–6 Hz spike-wave complexes. This subsyndrome accounted for 23% of all JME cases in the authors' dataset.

The fourth subsyndrome of JME starts with myoclonic seizures and grand mal convulsions during adolescence and pyknoleptic absences follow after 18 years of age. This fourth subsyndrome accounted for 5% of all JME cases in the authors' dataset.

The subsyndromes of JME mixed with childhood and adolescent pyknoleptic absences have multiplex and multigenerational families in 40% of pedigrees studied. Grand mal, myoclonias and absences appear in affected members. The segregation ratio across all matings is 0.17 and 0.31 across normal by affected matings.

The authors' laboratories have genotyped families with the subsyndrome of classic JME and have found one chromosome locus in 6p. They are presently mapping the chromosomal loci of JME mixed with pyknoleptic absences.

CLASSIC JME

Initial proof for linkage to chromosome 6p

At the Lafora Neurological Society meetings in Madrid in 1986 and at the Human Gene Mapping 9 Workshop in 1987, the authors' team reported for the first time the existence of an epilepsy gene by showing that classic JME without pyknoleptic absences may be linked to the Bf-HLA loci in chromosome 6p (Greenberg *et al.*, 1988). Using clinical and EEG characteristics of affected family members, their laboratories reported a pooled maximum LOD score of 3.04 at recombination fractions of $\theta_m = 0.01$ and $\theta_f = 0.10$ under a recessive model of inheritance assuming full penetrance using HLA and Bf (properdin factor) as markers. They obtained these results from 24 nuclear families, 11 of which were informative for Bf and three for HLA. Because they subsequently found no significant association with any specific alleles of HLA and because of one recombinant family, it was suggested that the JME locus may lie outside the HLA region. Evidence for possible linkage was strengthened when Greenberg *et al.* (1988) increased the original sample to 33 families: 18 were informative for Bf and four for HLA. The maximum LOD score obtained for this analysis was 3.78 ($\theta_{m=f} = 0.01$) assuming autosomal dominant (AD) inheritance and 90% penetrance. Assuming autosomal recessive (AR) inheritance with complete penetrance, the maximum LOD score was 3.05 ($\theta_{m=f} = 0.01$) (Greenberg *et al.*, 1987, 1988; Greenberg and Delgado-Escueta, 1993).

Independent proof of linkage to chromosome 6p in one large family (Figure 1)

In 1993 to 1994, the authors studied under the assumption of homogeneity 38 members of a four-generation LA-Belize family (J001) with classical JME but with no pyknoleptic absences (Liu *et al.*, 1995; Serratosa *et al.*, 1996). Five living members had JME and four clinically asymptomatic members had EEG multispike-wave complexes. Pairwise analysis tightly linked microsatellites centromeric to HLA, namely D6S272 (peak LOD score $Z_{max} = 3.564$–3.560 at male-female recombination ($\theta_{m=f} = 0.01$) and D6S257 ($Z_{max} = 3.672$–3.6667 at $\theta_{m=f} = 0.001$), spanning 7 cM, to convulsive seizures and EEG multispike-wave complexes. A recombination between D6S276 and D6S273 in one affected member placed the JME locus within or below HLA. Pairwise, multipoint, and recombination analyses in this large family independently proved that a JME gene is located in chromosome 6p, centromeric to HLA.

Classic JME in 6p: extension of linkage study to small multiplex families

Using the same chromosome 6p21.2-p11 short tandem-repeat polymorphic markers, the authors' laboratories then screened seven multiplex pedigrees with classic JME. When LOD scores for small multiplex families are added to LOD scores of the LA-Belize pedigree, Z_{max} values for D6S294 and D6S257 are >7 at $\theta_{m=f} = 0.00$. These results proved that in chromosome 6p21.2-p11 an epilepsy locus exists whose phenotype consists of classic JME with convulsions and/or EEG rapid multispike-wave complexes (Liu *et al.*, 1995).

Multipoint analysis and recombinations in small and large families with classic JME in 6p

In 1996, multipoint analysis and recombinations in three additional but small families from Mexico and Los Angeles, USA, narrowed the JME 6p locus to a 6 cM interval flanked by D6S272 and D6S257. Since the conditional

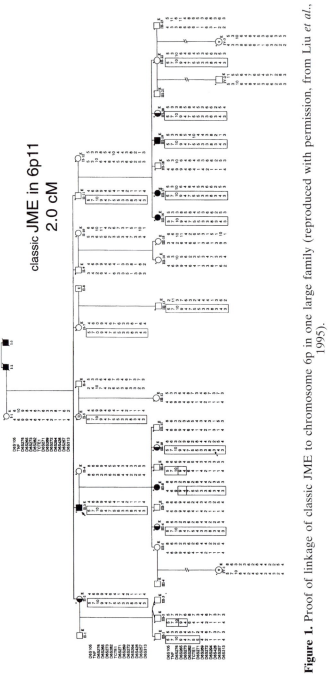

Figure 1. Proof of linkage of classic JME to chromosome 6p in one large family (reproduced with permission, from Liu *et al.*, 1995).

probability of linkage is a useful way of identifying families that may be linked, the authors separated those families whose posterior probabilities of linkage were larger than 0.60. Assuming AD inheritance with 70% penetrance, nine markers were observed, namely TCTE1, D6S271, D6S282, D6S272, D6S466, D6S294, D6S257, D6S402 and D6S430, showing significant Z_{max} (3.8–9.1 at $\theta_{m=f} = 0.00$–0.10) for these 11 families. Exclusionary LOD scores (−14.742 to −1.364; at $\theta_{m=f} = 0.00$ to 0.05) were obtained for TNF. These eleven markers (D6S89, D6S105, TNF, TCTE1, D6S271, D6S272, D6S466, D6S294, D6S257, D6S402, D6S430) were then used for multipoint linkage analysis in 11 linked families. The genetic distance between STRPs used were based on the genetic linkage map published by Genethon (Gyapay et al., 1994). The LOD score curve led to the highest peak value of 14.576 between D6S466 and D6S294, a 2 cM interval. According to the ($Z_{max} - 1$) method, the JME locus is probably in the region spanned by D6S272-(D6S466–D6S294)–D6S257, a 6 cM space (Liu et al., 1996).

Most recently, the authors reviewed all informative recombinations, which had previously been identified in our linked JME families. Because the distance is measured between D6S466 and D6S465 as 4 Mb based on our YACs, the JME region is calculated flanked by D6S294 and D6S465 to measure conservatively 6 Mb. A recombination between TNF and TCTE1 in one affected member (family 68-9) agrees with the previously observed recombination in the LA-Belize family (J001), suggesting a JME region below TNF. A recombination between D6S426 and TCTE1 in two affected members (family 170-30 and 170-2) placed the JME region below D6S426, which is 11 cM below HLA.

Recombinations in five clinically affected individuals of family 106 place the JME region in a 6 cM interval flanked by D6S465 telomeric and D6S294 centromeric.

Heterogeneity in JME: non-6p-linked families are JME mixed with pyknoleptic absences

The authors next explored whether the same chromosome 6p11 microsatellites also have a role in small families with JME mixed with pyknoleptic absences and allow for heterogeneity during analyses (Liu et al., 1996). Heterogeneity was tested for by the admixture test and looked for more recombinations. D6S272, D6S466, D6S294 and D6S257 were significantly linked ($Z_{max} > 3.5$) to the clinical and EEG traits of 22 families whose probands have JME with or without pyknoleptic absences, assuming AD inheritance with 70% penetrance. Pairwise Z_{max} values were 4.230 for D6S294 ($\theta_{m=f}$ at 0.133) and 4.442 for D6S466 ($\theta_{m=f}$ at 0.111). The admixture test (H_2 versus H_1) was significant ($p = 0.0234$ for D6S294 and 0.0128 for D6S272) supporting the hypotheses of linkage with heterogeneity. Estimated proportion of linked families was

$\alpha = 0.50$ (95% confidence interval 0.05–0.99) for D6S294 and D6S272. Phenotype analyses showed families linked to 6p were classic JME while families not linked to 6p were JME mixed with pyknoleptic absences (Liu *et al.*, 1996).

JME MIXED WITH PYKNOLEPTIC CHILDHOOD ABSENCES OR PYKNOLEPTIC CAE EVOLVING TO JME IN CHROMOSOME 1p

Because non-6p-linked families had phenotypes of JME mixed with pyknoleptic absences, families were recruited with such phenotypes for genome wide screens. When the phenotypes of all probands ascertained as JME are analysed, pyknoleptic absences appear in late childhood in 27%, in adolescence in 23% and after 18 years in 5%. When all probands ascertained as pyknoleptic childhood absence epilepsy are analysed, about 10–12% evolve into JME. Put another way, one subsyndrome of childhood absences starts between 5 and 10 years of age as frequent daily flurries of absences, much like classic childhood pyknoleptic absences, but myoclonic seizures and grand mal convulsions appear during adolescence, making it difficult to distinguish from JME. Such patients' EEGs also show irregular spike- and polyspike-wave complexes in addition to classic or typical 3 Hz spike- and slow-wave complexes during absences. Mai *et al.* (1990) estimate 5.3% and Janz (1985) mentions 4.6% of JME evolves out of childhood pyknoleptic absences.

One large family (M17), from Mexico City and Guadalajara, was studied whose affected members had pyknoleptic absences (childhood- or adolescent-onset) only, or absence plus grand mal convulsions, or JME or grand mal seizures only. The family was ascertained through a proband with pyknoleptic childhood absence and typical 3 Hz spike-waves and also irregular polyspike-waves. During adolescence she developed grand mal convulsions and myoclonias. In other words, her illness had evolved into JME. After performing EEGs in 109 family members, 43 members belonging to three generations were initially genotyped of whom six members were considered affected in all analyses. Affected members had either juvenile absences only (female cousin), grand mal only (brother), absence with grand mal (grandmother, mother, female cousin) or JME (female cousin). One female cousin (member no. 50) was asymptomatic but had typical 3 Hz spike- and multispike-waves. In addition, two first-degree male cousins had partial seizures of temporal lobe origin and one has cysticercosis.

In 1996, Westling *et al.* (1996), Westling (1997) and Gee *et al.* (unpublished data) observed significant linkage in this family. Westling *et al.* performed sib pair analyses of 286 polymorphic DNA markers located throughout the genome using the SAGE program SIBPAL and then model-based linkage analyses of the 22 markers of interest. Five markers (D1S448, D1S550,

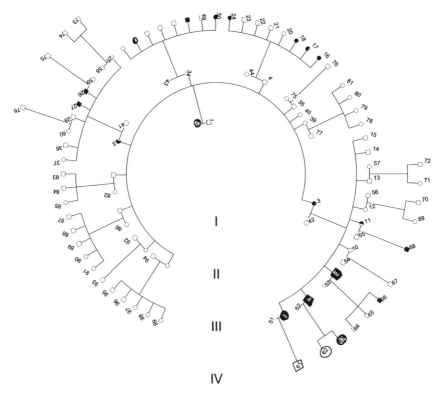

Figure 2. Study of four generations of one family to reveal evidence of genetic linkage of JME mixed with pyknoleptic childhood absences or pyknoleptic CAE evolving to JME to chromosome 1p.

D1S500, D1S465, D1S207) showed indications of linkage ($p <0.01$) and were within approximately 7 cM on chromosome 1p. D1S305 showed positive scores when members affected with partial epilepsies were considered affected. D1S305 is 34 cM centromeric to the cluster of markers that showed significant scores. Other markers which showed significance ($p <0.01$) were D2S427, D9S303, D12S61 and D21S156. Evidence for linkage for marker D1S207 disappeared when members with 'partial epilepsies' or member 50 were considered affected. The strongest evidence for linkage was obtained for D2S427 ($p <0.00005$ under all definitions).

Westling and Weissbecker (unpublished data) subsequently analysed 22 markers of interest using an AD inheritance model with 70% penetrance and a narrow diagnostic model that considered members with partial epilepsy and member 50 as unaffected. They obtained the best LOD score of 3.8 for D1S207. Multipoint analysis showed 3.803 LOD score when the epilepsy locus was directly at D1S207. One recombination between the epilepsy and D1S550, D1S465 and D1S448 suggested that the epilepsy gene is centromeric to these markers at or below D1S207 and D1S488. Using the Bonferroni correction for multiple testing (Risch, 1991; Lander and Schork, 1994) where LOD score after it is increased by log 10(k) is 3.78, the score of 3.799 obtained for D1S207 remained significant (Westling *et al.*, 1996, Westling, 1997 and unpublished data).

However, the first cousin with 3 Hz spike-waves raises the question whether genetic linkage to chromosome 1p is truly present. For this reason, this family has now been extended to 28 more members including 14 members of the fourth generation (Figure 2). Their EEGs have been completed and four EEG-affected members (3–5 Hz spike-waves) in the third generation and three members with epilepsies in the fourth generation (one with childhood absences that evolved to JME, two with grand mal seizures only) have been identified. Twelve medium-sized families with the same syndrome are also being studied.

PHOTOGENIC CHILDHOOD ABSENCES WITH EYELID MYOCLONIAS EVOLVING TO JME

Another dilemma in the diagnosis of JME is photogenic pyknoleptic absences with eyelid myoclonia that develop into grand mal and myoclonic seizures during late childhood or adolescence consistent with the diagnosis of JME. Affected members are mostly females. Absence seizures may be self-induced. First reported by Radovici *et al.* in 1932, and by Andermann *et al.* in 1962, this syndrome is also called eyelid myoclonia with absences by Jeavons *et al.*, (1972) and Jeavons and Hardin (1975). Panayiotopoulos *et al.* (1989) and Panayiotopoulos (1994) describe its key features as (1) eye-closure-induced eyelid myoclonia with absences starting during childhood with grand mal tonic-clonic seizures developing in adult life; half also have myoclonic seizures; (2) photosensitivity, and (3) 3–6 Hz polyspike-waves triggered by eye closure and eliminated in darkness.

Because the majority of affected family members have JME (adolescent onset myoclonias only or with grand mal seizures) or absences with eyelid myoclonia, myoclonic and grand mal seizures, the authors favour considering them as a clinical subsyndrome of JME.

A 133-member multiplex-multigenerational family (LA40) was identified through a proband whose pyknoleptic absences started at three years of age, associated with eyelid myoclonia. CCTV-EEG telemetry caught her inducing absences by looking at the sun and waving the outstretched fingers of her hands in front of the sunlight (Andermann *et al.*, 1962). Between eight and ten years of age, tonic clonic convulsions started. At 12 years, myoclonic seizures were more frequent. Four members of her family are affected electroencephalographically with spike-wave discharges and myoclonias during photic stimulation but are otherwise clinically asymptomatic. History showed that 13 other family members are affected clinically, six of whom have JME. These include spontaneous or photic-induced myoclonias and grand mal seizures that started at 11 years of age (sister and mother), or myoclonic seizures only (two cousins), or childhood absences that persisted with grand mal and myoclonic seizures during adolescence (two cousins). Other seizure types were childhood absence plus grand mal (two cousins); childhood absence only (two cousins); and grand mal only (three cousins). EEG and photic stimulation demonstrated pyknoleptic absences with 2.5–3.5 Hz spike waves with eyelid myoclonia and myoclonic seizures with 5–15 Hz rapid spikes in nine of these 13 patients. Eleven members were female and two male (one with absence and one with myoclonias.)

Sixty-five family members were screened with the sixth version of the Weber laboratory screening set which consists of 169 microsatellites with average heterozygosity of 0.78 and an average spacing of 24.2 cM. LOD scores of more than 1.5 at $\theta = 0$ identified four chromosomal regions, namely 1p, 2p, 12p and 19q (Delgado-Escueta et al., 1999) and these areas are now being studied with more markers.

THE SYNDROME OF CHILDHOOD ABSENCE EPILEPSY

To succeed in linkage analysis and mapping, it is important to separate the syndrome of typical childhood absence epilepsy from the syndromes of pyknoleptic absences that evolve to JME. The GENES international consortium separated four subsyndromes within 120 families with childhood absence epilepsies. The first subsyndrome is the classic self-remitting pyknoleptic childhood absence epilepsy that starts between 5 and 10 years of age with multiple petit mal seizures (1–200 per day) during regular bilaterally symmetrical and synchronous 3 Hz spike waves. Petit mal absences remit or disappear in a quarter of cases by 16–20 years of age and in three-quarters of cases by 30 years of age (Gibberd, 1966). Neither myoclonias nor grand mal tonic-clonic seizures ever develop. This self-remitting subsyndrome accounts for 57% of the authors' patients. It has been reported to account for 33% (Oller-Daurella and Sanchez, 1981) to 57% (Loiseau et al., 1983) of all childhood absences. The second subsyndrome also starts as flurries of pyknoleptic absences between 5 and 10 years of age but grand mal convulsions soon develop in late childhood or adolescence. The EEG shows irregular 3–6 Hz spikes and polyspike- and slow-wave complexes. No myoclonic seizures develop but the epilepsies persist into adulthood. This second subsyndrome, persisting childhood pyknoleptic absence epilepsy, is a

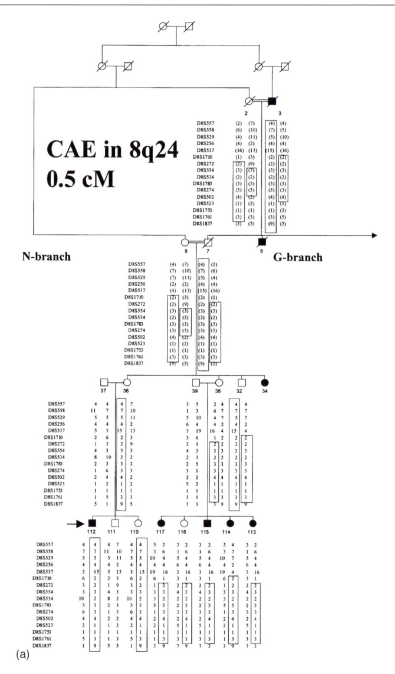

Figure 3. (a) and (b) Proof of linkage of typical childhood absence epilepsy to chromosome 8q24 in a large Indian family.

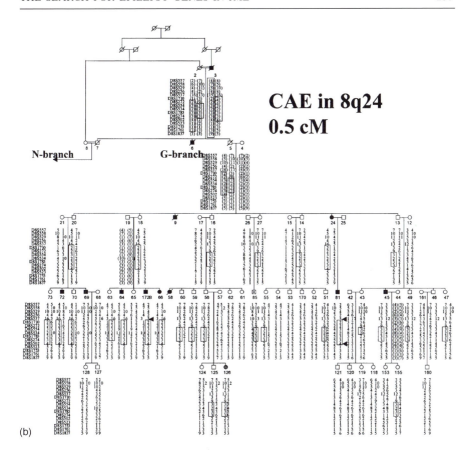

(b)

common subsyndrome in the authors' dataset and accounts for 28% of all patients. It is estimated to account for 40% (Loiseau *et al.*, 1983) to 60% (Oller-Daurella and Sanchez, 1981) of all childhood absence epilepsies. The third subsyndrome of childhood absences also starts between 5 and 10 years of age but evolves into JME since myoclonic seizures and grand mal convulsions appear during adolescence. The EEG shows irregular spike- and polyspike-wave complexes. In this third subsyndrome, the patient is also afflicted with many flurries of absences, much like classic childhood pyknoleptic absences, but myoclonias and grand mal convulsions develop during adolescence and persist well into mature and old age. Mai *et al.* (1990) estimates 5.3% and Janz (1985) mentions that 4.6% of JME evolves out of childhood pyknoleptic absences. The authors estimate that this third subsyndrome accounts for 10–12% of all childhood absences. The fourth subsyndrome consists of photogenic CAE with eyelid myoclonia that evolves to JME. This constitutes about 3% of all CAE syndromes. The authors believe that the typical CAE syndromes may or may not remit and may or may not have accompanying tonic-clonic seizures, but that they should not involve myoclonic seizures. Otherwise they belong to the JME syndromes.

INDEPENDENT PROOF FOR LINKAGE IN ONE LARGE FAMILY WITH TYPICAL CHILDHOOD ABSENCE EPILEPSY IN CHROMOSOME 8q24

A large family from Bombay, India

The GENES international consortium obtained independent proof for linkage to chromosome 8q24 microsatellites in a large, multiplex, multigeneration family from Bombay, India (I201) (Fong *et al.*, 1998). This family was ascertained through a 17-year-old patient with pyknoleptic childhood absences, as described originally by Adie (1924) and Calmeil (1824), grand mal seizures and electroencephalographic regular and irregular 3–4 Hz spike- and multispike-wave complexes, as described by Gibbs *et al.* (1935). Clinical examination and EEGs were performed in 78 family members, 11 of whom were affected either with absences and/or 3–4 Hz spike- and multispike-wave complexes only (six members) or absences with grand mal (five members) (Figures 3(a) and 3(b)). The clinical states of three other affected members were assessed as secondary generalized seizures with partial onset. One of these members had exclusively nocturnal seizures and centrotemporal sharp waves, as described by Bray and Wiser (1964, 1965) and was suspected to have Rolandic epilepsy, as described by Beaussart (1972) and Beaussart and Faou (1978). Three persons had febrile seizures that could have other genotypes or causes besides the childhood absence syndrome. Hence, these were considered unaffected for linkage analyses.

Linkage analysis tested two diagnostic models. In the first, narrow diagnostic model, only family members who have childhood pyknoleptic absences, typical 3 Hz spike-wave complexes and grand mal tonic-clonic seizures were classified as affected. In a second, broad diagnostic model, individuals with other forms of epilepsy such as partial epilepsies evolving to secondary generalized epilepsies, including Rolandic epilepsy, were also classified as affected. Beaumanoir *et al.* (1974) originally observed that Rolandic spikes could appear in a person with absences and spike-wave paroxysms.

Segregation of the absence phenotype followed an AD mode with incomplete penetrance (Metrakos and Metrakos, 1961a, 1961b, 1966, 1969).

The authors first pursued the hypothesis that an epilepsy locus was in one of three chromosomal sites, namely 1p or 6p or 8q24. The Affected Pedigree Member method (APM) multilocus analyses (Weeks and Lange, 1988) showed significant *p*-values (0.00003), suggesting linkage to D8S256, D8S272, D8S534, D8S274 and D8S502, all located in chromosome 8q24. Two-point linkage analysis, assuming an AD model of inheritance with 50% penetrance, and testing the narrow diagnostic model for absence epilepsy and/or 3–4 Hz spike-wave complexes, yielded a LOD score of 3.7 for D8S502 at $\theta_{m=f} = 0.00$. In the broad diagnostic model (all forms of epilepsies including partial epilepsies and febrile convulsions considered affected), the highest LOD score for D8S502 was 2.44 at ($\theta_{m=f} = 0.00$) under AD inheritance with 50% penetrance. When only the person with Rolandic epilepsy together with family members with absences and EEG 3–4 Hz spike-waves were considered, the LOD score was still below 3.0. A genome-wide screen looking for other major susceptibility loci using another 169 markers was also carried out and found no other loci with major effects comparable to 8q24 that also fulfilled the standard for significant linkage.

Recombinations place the CAE locus in a 0.5 cM area

Recombinant events in three affected members (nos 117, 115, 114, 113) placed the gene locus in a 5.7 cM region flanked centromerically by D8S537 and telomerically by D8S1837 in 8q24. A recombination in members 114, 172B and 8 cut the centromeric border to D8S1710; member 172B also cut the telomeric border to D8S502, making the flanking markers D8S1710 (centromere) and D8S502 (telomere) for the 3.2 cM CAE interval. After consanguinity and assortative matings in the first and second generation were recognized, it was possible to follow the haplotypes segregate down to affected members of the fifth generation. This reduced the critical region further to 0.5 cM.

Extension of linkage study to small multiplex families with typical CAE

Analysis was extended to five smaller multiplex families with the same syndrome and screened with same 8q24 microsatellites. Positive LOD scores were obtained for D8S537 (LOD score = 2.4), and D8S1761 (LOD score = 1.7) at $\theta = 0$. Haplotypes segregated in all five families with affected members. Informative recombinations in three families (S302, S2 and LA112) placed CAE in a region flanked by D8S1710 and D8S502.

Three separate epilepsy loci probably exist in chromosome 8q. The first locus reported by Lewis et al. (1993) was genetically heterogenous and was demonstrated in one Mexican-American family with BFNC that showed tight linkage to chromosome 8q. Multipoint analysis placed the gene locus (EBN2) between D8S198 and D8S274. This syndrome has now been shown to be associated with a mutation in the KCNQ3 channel gene (Charlier et al., 1998).

The second locus was reported by Zara et al. (1995) who studied idiopathic generalized epilepsy families from Italy by parametric and nonparametric methods of linkage analysis. This study mixed together five families with childhood absence epilepsy, two families with juvenile myoclonic epilepsy, one family with grand mal epilepsy and two families with febrile seizures. In four of these families, different idiopathic generalized epilepsy syndromes occured in members of the same family. In spite of these mixtures of disparate epilepsy syndromes, highly significant results were obtained with marker D8S256, initially with the extended sib pair analysis and then with the affected pedigree member method.

The third report suggesting an epilepsy locus in chromosome 8q came from Wallace *et al.* (1996) who studied one large Australian family where many individuals had febrile convulsions and the most severely affected had temporal lobe epilepsy with hippocampal scleroses. Linkage to chromosome 8q13-21 was considered only suggestive because LOD scores did not reach the threshhold for significance, namely 3.0.

The chromosome 8q24 locus, which the authors reported for the childhood absence syndrome (Gee *et al.*, 1997; Fong *et al.*, 1998) is approximately 5 cM telomeric to EBN2 or the second genotype for benign familial neonatal convulsions. It is also about 5 cM telomeric from the region Zara *et al.* (1995) suspected was the susceptibility locus for idiopathic generalized epilepsies. The chromosome 8q13 locus of the Australian family with febrile seizures (Wallace *et al.*, 1996) seems quite distant and more centromeric from the 8q24 locus which the present authors' have defined for absence epilepsy (Gee *et al.*, 1997; Fong *et al.*, 1998).

DISCUSSION

Using large families to look for the 'Janz gene'

Lander and Schork (1994) stated, 'in linkage analyses, the simplest situation is when unequivocal linkage can be demonstrated in a single large pedigree (with lod score more than 3 or more than 4 depending on the number of tests performed)'. Thus, between 1993 and 1996, the present authors concentrated their efforts on mapping epilepsy genes in large multiplex families and then extending their studies to smaller multiplex families, seeking confirmation of linkage. Rigorous evidence was sought from independent datasets from different countries before positional cloning was undertaken to avoid the unpleasant task of chasing a phantom locus. Each of the large families from Belize (JME), Mexico (JME and JME mixed with absences), India (CAE), Palestine (Lafora's disease), the Appalachian mountains of Kentucky, USA (Lafora's disease) and California, USA (CAE with eyelid myoclonia evolving to JME) provided independent proof for linkage to an epilepsy syndrome. In each family, more than three markers were found in each of chromosomes 6p11, 1p, 8q24, 6q24 and 12p, respectively, that yielded LOD scores higher than 3.3, the asymptotic threshold corresponding to

Bonferroni corrections for the number of tests performed, and higher than 3.6 or $p = 2 \times 10^{-5}$, the genome-wide significance level or the 5% chance of finding a region as extreme as 2×10^{-5}.

Is the chromosome 6p epilepsy gene within HLA or below HLA? Or, are there two epilepsy genes in 6p, one within HLA and one below HLA?

In 1991, Weissbecker *et al.*, in a replication study of the JME gene, analysed 23 families from Berlin, Germany, and confirmed the linkage to 6p, and excluded *tight* linkage to HLA. Weissbecker *et al.* agreed with the present authors' original suggestions in 1988 that the JME gene is outside the HLA region. They reported summed LOD scores of 3.11 ($\theta_m = 0.001$ and $\theta_f = 0.20$) in 23 small families from Berlin, assuming AD inheritance. Also, in 1991, Durner *et al.*, from the Free University of Berlin, collaborated with Greenberg (who had moved to New York) and used the same Berlin families reported by Weissbecker *et al.* (1991) and reported tight linkage to DNA markers in the HLA-DQ locus. Tight linkage was not as evident (Z_{max} of 4.1 but with $\theta_m = 0.01$ and $\theta_f = 0.3$) when asymptomatic members with EEG multispike-wave complexes were considered affected. Sander *et al.* (1997a) recently updated linkage studies in families from Germany. They again showed significant LOD scores for chromosome 6p microsatellites and observed five recombinations that locate the JME locus approximately 10 cM below HLA-DR. This agrees with our results that the JME gene is below HLA. However, these results are some 10 cM away from Sander *et al*'s published data since we locate the critical region at 19–25 cM below and centromeric to HLA. These studies from Berlin and Los Angeles, reporting recombinations in small families of JME, could miscalculate the exact distance of the JME gene below HLA. With the exception of the large Belize family (Liu *et al.*, 1996 and Serratosa *et al.*, 1996), none of the JME families from Berlin and Austria (Sander *et al.*, 1997) and Los Angeles and Mexico (Liu *et al.*, 1996) have individual LOD scores that reach significance. Studies in small families, whose individual LOD scores do not reach significance, should be interpreted with caution because heterogeneity exists in JME. Some, if not many, of these small families may not be truly linked to chromosome 6p and the suggested recombinations could be misleading.

In 1996, Greenberg and his collaborators in New York suggested that the JME locus resides within the HLA region, most likely between HLA-DP and HLA-B loci (Greenberg *et al.*, 1996). This argument would make the EJM1 locus distinct from the epilepsy locus, which our group (Liu *et al.*, 1995, 1996; Serratosa *et al.*, 1996) and the Berlin group (Sander *et al.*, 1997) claim is some 10–30 cM below HLA in chromosome 6p. Greenberg *et al.* (1996) studied HLA-DR and DQ frequencies in 24 JME patients and in 24 non-JME forms of adolescent-onset idiopathic generalized epilepsies from New York. The frequency of DR13 and DQB1 alleles was significantly higher in JME. Durner *et al.* (1992) also reported a weak association with the HLA-DRw6 allele (odds ratio of 2.5). DRw6 was split into two antigens, DR13 and DR14. In 1994, Obeid *et al.* also noted that DR13 was associated with JME in families from Saudi Arabia with an odds ratio of 4.5 (Obeid and Panayiotopoulos, 1988; Panayiatopolous and Obeid, 1989). Thus, these three HLA association studies, by Greenberg *et al.* (1996), Durner *et al.* (1991) and Obeid *et al.* (1994) suggest that a second epilepsy gene may be present in chromosome 6p, lying within the HLA complex. JME families from Los Angeles, Belize, Mexico and Germany have not shown significant association with HLA alleles (Liu *et al.*, 1995, Serratosa *et al.*, 1996, Sander *et al.*, 1997).

Locus heterogeneity in JME (Table 1)

Aside from the authors' studies, evidence for heterogeneity in JME was reported in 1992 and 1996 by Gardiner's group using 25 JME families from the UK and Sweden (Elmslie *et al.*, 1996). Results excluded linkage to chromosome 6p markers suggesting heterogeneity. In 1997, Elmslie *et al.* presented data supporting a second JME locus in chromosome 15q using the same UK and Swedish families that have JME with absences.

In 1995 and 1997, Pandolfo and collaborators from the Italian League Against Epilepsy reported two separate putative susceptibility loci for idiopathic generalized epilepsies, namely, grand mal and generalized spike-waves in chromosome 3p (Zara *et al.*, 1997) and generalized epilepsies and EEG spike-waves in 8q24 (Zara *et al.*, 1995). Some of the families reported to link to 8q24 have the JME phenotype.

Candidate genes for the JME syndrome of Janz and typical CAE

At the present time, three serious candidate genes have been studied in families with JME or CAE.

The first candidate gene that is presently being studied in families with JME in 6p is the GABA-B receptor gene (Kaupmann *et al.*, 1997), located within the lower limits of the chromosome 6p HLA area. Theoretically, this is an excellent candidate for mutations in JME families from Los Angeles (Greenberg *et al.*, 1988), New York (Greenberg *et al.*, 1996) and Berlin (Durner *et al.*, 1991) that have been reported to be linked to the HLA region. GABA, the principal inhibitory neurotransmitter, signals through ionotropic (GABA-A) and metabotropic (GABA-B) receptor systems. Metabotropic receptors couple to G proteins and modulate synaptic transmission through intracellular effector systems. GABA-B receptors have received much attention in absence seizures because microinjections of agonists (baclofen) and

antagonists (CGP 35348) into the nucleus ventralis thalami, nucleus reticularis thalami, and nucleus reuniens enhance or suppress absences through the
oscillatory and reverberating thalamocortical circuits in the lethargic mice
model for absences (Hosford et al., 1992, 1995). GABA-B anatagonists
systemically administered in absence rats from Strasbourg (Marescaux et al.,
1992) and in pharmacologic models of absence seizures (Snead, 1994)
produced the same results.

Kaupmann et al. (1997) recently identified cDNAs which encode two
GABA-B receptor proteins designated GABA-bR1a and bR1b. The human
GABA-B receptor (HGABABR) was cloned by cDNA hybridization selection and mapped to 6p21.3. However, Choi et al. (1998) failed to detect any
mutations in HGABABR in patients with JME. They used single-stranded
conformational polymorphism (SSCP) and base excision sequencing scanning
(BESS) to screen for mutations in 11 dyslexic patients and nine JME
patients. Polymorphisms were detected but no mutations segregated with
affected members with either dyslexia or JME. Further studies, however,
need to be made of patients who belong to families that show linkage to
chromosome 6p. We know that there is locus heterogeneity in JME, and
Choi et al. (1998) did not study families that showed linkage to JME; they
merely studied JME patients whose chromosome locus was not known.
Sander et al. (1997) also analysed the relationship between idiopathic generalized epilepsies and GABA-A receptor alpha5, beta3 and gamma3 subunit
gene cluster on chromosome 15 and found no clear evidence of genetic
linkage.

A second candidate gene that still has to be ruled out in JME is the human
jerky gene in chromosome 6p. In 1995, Toth et al. reported an insertional
murine mutation that inactivated a novel gene and resulted in whole body
jerks, generalized clonic seizures, and epileptic brain activity in transgenic
mice. The insertion of the transgene is accompanied by a deletion of a 9 kb
DNA sequence including the coding region of the cellular gene. Because of
the characteristic whole body jerking during seizures, Toth et al. named the
locus and the gene 'jerky'. The murine gene, called jerky, encodes a putative
41.7 kD protein displaying homology to a number of nuclear regulatory
proteins, suggesting that perhaps the jerky protein is able to bind DNA.
These authors (Toth et al., 1995) further defined the approximately 8 kb
jerky gene which contains multiple exons. DNA sequencing of the murine
jerky gene revealed an open reading frame encoding a putative 41.7 kb
protein of 370 amino acid residues in a single exon. Homozygotes for the
jerky gene display other abnormalities such as growth retardation, short life
span, and male sterility in addition to seizures. Jerky was mapped between
D15Mit3 and the retrovirus integration site, Pmv17/tef, on chromosome 15.

Zeng et al. (1997) and the authors' collaborators, Morita et al. (1998)
mapped the human homologue of the murine jerky gene to chromosomes

6p21 (JH6), 8q24 (JH8) and 11p21-23 (JH11). The JH6 or the human jerky gene in 6p is an excellent candidate gene for the epilepsy syndrome of JME, especially because FISH locates its sequences in 6p21. Zeng *et al.* (1997) obtained all cDNA clones corresponding to the human jerky gene from ESTs. cDNA clones corresponding to the human jerky gene that maps to chromosome 6p21 is approximately 70 kb and contains mainly exon coding regions with its open reading frame calculated to be about 40 kb, containing 3000 nucleotides coding for a protein that has 470 amino acids. The authors' laboratories have yet to screen for mutations in JH6 gene in JME families from Los Angeles that show tight linkage to HLA.

However, the authors' team did rule out JH8 as the site of mutations in families with CAE. JH8 had been considered a good candidate for the CAE mutation because this human jerky gene also maps to chromosome 8q24. FISH and radiation hybrid show its location at the telomeric end of the critical region for CAE in 8q24 (Morita *et al.*, 1998). Mutation analyses of the JH8 gene revealed seven nucleotide changes, including amino acid substitutions that did not segregate with the disease phenotype of CAE (Morita *et al.*, 1998).

The potassium channel gene of the long Q-T family (KvLQT) named KCNQ3 which maps to the centromeric end of the CAE 8q24 locus can be ruled out as the site of mutations for the Bombay, Saudi Arabia, Spanish, Argentina and USA families with CAE. Submicroscopic microdeletion, missense, frameshift and splice site mutations for benign familial neonatal convulsions in 20q and a missense mutation for the same phenotype in 8q24 had been defined to reside in the voltage-sensitive potassium channel belonging to the long Q-T family, dubbed KCNQ2 and KCNQ3, respectively (Singh *et al.*, 1998, Charlier *et al.*, 1998). KCNQ2 and KCNQ3 share about 70% amino acid identity with the KCNQ1 gene that is responsible for the AD long Q-T syndrome of cardiac arrhythmia of Romano-Ward syndrome and the AR Jervell and Lange-Nielsen syndrome of deafness and long Q-T syndrome (Sanguinneti *et al.*, 1996). However, KCNQ3 is about 5 cM away from the CAE 8q24 locus. Moreover, no amino acid sequence changes in KCNQ3 segregate with the CAE phenotypes in families from Bombay, Riyahd, and Madrid.

ACKNOWLEDGEMENTS

We wish to acknowledge some of our many colleagues who participate as part of the GENES international consortium. Our accomplishments and successes in recruiting families and mapping epilepsy genes would not have been possible without their participation and contributions. Specifically, we wish to mention Dr Jose M. Serratosa (now directing the Epilepsy Unit,

Service of Neurology, Fundacion Jimenez Diaz, Madrid, Spain), Dr Pravina Shah and her team (Neurology Department, KEM Hospital, Bombay, India), Dr Ignacio Pascual-Castroviejo (Pediatric Neurology, University Hospital La Paz, Madrid, Spain), Dr Sergio Cordova (previously at the National Institute of Neurology and Neurosurgery, Mexico City, Mexico) and Dr Sonia Khan (Department of Neurosciences, Military Hospital, Riyadh, Saudi Arabia). These colleagues, along with others in California (especially Dr Gregorio Pineda, Bakersfield, and Dr Gregory Walsh, Santa Monica), have referred and enrolled patients as part of the GENES international consortium. Others have played an important role as neuroscientists (Lucy M. Treiman, Ph.D. and Jesus Sainz, Ph.D.), geneticists (Robert Sparkes, Ph.D.), co-ordinators (Joan Spellman, Adriana Lopez, Bernadette Sakamoto, Susan Pietsch), neurologists (Dr Berge Minassian, Dr Surisham Dhillon), laboratory technicians (Aurelio Jara Prado, Susan Shih, Reza Iranmanesh) and EEG technicians (Nancy Kjeldgaard and Charlotte McTerrell).

REFERENCES

Adie, W.J. (1924). Pyknolepsy: a form of epilepsy occurring in children with a good prognosis. *Brain* **47**, 96–102.

Andermann, K., Oaks, G., Berman, S. *et al.* (1962). Self-induced epilepsy. *Arch Neurol* **6**, 49–79.

Beaumanoir, A., Ballis, T., Warfis, G. and Ansari, K. (1974). Benign epilepsy of childhood with rolandic spikes. *Epilepsia* **15**, 301–315.

Beaussart, M. (1972). Benign epilepsy of children with Rolandic centro-temporal paroxysmal foci: a clinical entity. Study of 221 cases. *Epilepsia* **13**, 793–796.

Beaussart, M. and Faou, R. (1978). Evolution of epilepsy with Rolandic paroxysmal foci: a study of 324 cases. *Epilepsia* **19**, 337–342.

Berkovic, S.F., Howell, R.A. and Hopper, J.L. (1994). Familial temporal lobe epilepsy: a new syndrome with adolescent/adult onset and a benign course. In: Wolf, P. (Ed.), *Epileptic Seizures and Syndromes*. John Libbey, London, pp. 257–263.

Berkovic, S.F., McIntosh, A.M., Howell, R.A., Mitchell, A., Sheffield, L.J. and Hopper, J.L. (1996). Familial temporal lobe epilepsy: a common disorder identified in twins. *Ann Neurol* **40**, 227–235.

Bray, P.F. and Wiser, W.C. (1964). Evidence for a genetic etiology of temporal-central abnormalities in focal epilepsy. *N Engl J Med* **271**, 926–933.

Bray, P.F. and Wiser, W.C. (1965). The relation of focal to diffuse epileptiform EEG discharges in genetic epilepsy. *Arch Neurol* **13**, 222–238.

Busard, H.L.S.M., Gobreels-Festen, A.A.W.M., Renih, W.U., Gabreels, F.J. and Stadhouders, A.M. (1987). Axilla skin biopsy; a reliable test for the diagnosis of Lafora's disease. *Ann Neurol* **21**, 599–601.

Calmeil, L.F. (1824). *De l'épilepsie, étudiée sous le rapport de son siège et de son influence sur la production de l'aliénation mentale.* [Thesis]. Paris.

Carpenter, S. and Karpati, G. (1981). Sweat gland duct cells in Lafora disease: diagnosis by skin biopsy. *Neurology* **31**, 1564–1568.

Castells, C. and Mendilaharsu, C. (1958). La epilepsia mioclonica bilateral y consciente. *Acta Neurol Latinoam* **4**, 23–48.

Charlier, C., Singh, N.A., Ryan, S.G. *et al.* (1998). A pore mutation in a novel KQT-like potassium channel gene in an idiopathic epilepsy family. *Nat Genet* **18**, 53–55.

Choi, J.J., Hisama, F.M., Gruen, J.R. *et al.* (1998). Mutation screening of the human GABA-B receptor gene in patients with juvenile myoclonic epilepsy and dyslexia [abstract]. *Am J Hum Genet* **63**, A356.

Commission on Classification and Terminology of the International League Against Epilepsy (1981). Proposal for revised clinical and electroencephalographic classification of epileptic seizures. *Epilepsia* **22**, 489–501.

Commission on Classification and Terminology of the International League Against Epilepsy (1989). Proposal for revised classification of epilepsies and epileptic syndromes. *Epilepsia* **30**, 389–399.

Delgado-Escueta, A.V. and Enrile-Bacsal, F.E. (1984). Juvenile myoclonic epilepsy of Janz. *Neurology* **34**, 285–294.

Delgado-Escueta, A.V., Fong, G.C.Y., Alonso, M.E. *et al.* (1999). Childhood absence epilepsy genotypes in chromosomes 8q24 and 1p: clinical and EEG phenotypes. 23rd International Epilepsy Congress.

Durner, M., Sander, T., Greenberg, D.A., Johnson, K., Beck-Mannagetta, G. and Janz, D. (1991). Localization of idiopathic generalized epilepsy on chromosome 6p in families of juvenile myoclonic epilepsy patients. *Neurology* **41**, 1651–1655.

Durner, M., Janz, D., Zingsem, J. and Greenberg, D.A. (1992). Possible association of juvenile myoclonic epilepsy with HLA-DRW6. *Epilepsia* **33**, 814–816.

Elmslie, F.V., Williamson, M.P., Rees, M. *et al.* (1996). Linkage analysis of juvenile myoclonic epilepsy and microsatellite loci spanning 61 cM of human chromosome 6p in 19 nuclear pedigrees provides no evidence for a susceptibility locus in this region. *Am J Hum Genet* **59**, 653–663.

Elmslie, F.V., Rees, M., Williamson, M.P. *et al.* (1997). Genetic mapping of a major susceptibility locus for juvenile myoclonic epilepsy on chromosome 15q. *Hum Mol Genet* **6**, 1329–1334.

Fong, G.C.Y., Shah, P.U., Gee, M.N. *et al.* (1998). Childhood absence epilepsy with tonic-clonic seizures and electroencephalogram 3–4 Hz spike and multispike-slow wave complexes: linkage to chromosome 8q24. *Am J Hum Genet* **63**, 1117–1129.

Gee, M.N., Huang, Y., Shah, P.U. *et al.* (1997). Childhood absence epilepsy: linkage to chromosome 8q24 [Poster]. Presented at the 122nd Annual Meeting of the American Neurological Association, San Diego, CA, 27 Sept–1 Oct.

Gibberd, F.B. (1966). The prognosis of petit mal. *Brain* **89**, 531–538.

Gibbs, F.A., Davis, H. and Lennox, W.G. (1935). The electro-encephalogram in epilepsy and in conditions of impaired consciousness. *Arch Neurol Psychiatry* **34**, 1133–1148.

Greenberg, D.A. and Delgado-Escueta, A.V. (1993). The chromosome 6p epilepsy locus: exploring mode of inheritance and heterogeneity through linkage analysis. *Epilepsia* **34** (suppl): 12–18.

Greenberg, D.A., Delgado-Escueta, A.V., Widelitz, H. *et al.* (1987). A locus involved in the expression of juvenile myoclonic epilepsy and of an associated EEG trait may be linked to HLA and Bf. *Cytogenet Cell Genet* **46**, 623.

Greenberg, D.A., Delgado-Escueta, A.V., Widelitz, H. *et al.* (1988). Juvenile myoclonic epilepsy (JME) may be linked to the Bf and HLA lock in human chromosome 6. *Am J Med Genet* **31**, 185–192.

Greenberg, D., Durner, M., Shinnar, S. *et al.* (1996). Association of HLA class II alleles in patients with juvenile myoclonic epilepsy compared to patients with other forms of adolescent-onset generalized epilepsy. *Neurology* **47**, 750–755.

Gyapay, G., Morissette, J., Vignal, J. *et al.* (1994). The 1993–1994 Genethon human genetic linkage map. *Nat Genet* **7**, 246–339.

Hauser, W.A. and Hesdorfer, D.C. (1990). *Epilepsy: Frequency, Causes and Consequences.* Demos.

Hosford, D.A., Clark, S., Cao, Z. *et al.* (1992). The role of GABA$_B$ receptor activation in absence seizures of lethargic (lh/lh) mice. *Science* **257**, 398–401.

Hosford, D.A., Link F.-H., Kraemer, D.L., Cao, Z., Wang, Y. and Wilson, J.T. (1995). Neural network of structures in which GABA$_B$ receptors regulate absence seizures in the lethargic (lh/lh) mouse model. *J Neurosci* **15**, 7367–7376.

Janz, D. (1969). *Die Epilepsien.* Thieme, Stuttgart, Germany.

Janz, D. (1985). Epilepsy with impulsive petit mal (juvenile myoclonic epilepsy). *Acta Neurol Scand* **72**, 449–459.

Janz, D. and Christian, W. (1957). Impulsiv-petit mal. *Dtsch Z Nervenheilk* **176**, 346–386.

Janz, D. and Matthes, A. (1955). *Die propulsiv petit mal Epilepsie.* Karger, New York.

Jeavons, P.M. and Hardin, G.F.A. (1975). *Photosensitive Epilepsy.* Heinemann, London.

Jeavons, P.M. Hardin, G.F.A., Panayiotopoulos, C.P. and Drasdo, N. (1972). The effect of geometric patterns combined with intermittent photic stimulation in photosensitive epilepsy. *Electroencephalogr Clin Neurophysiol* **33**, 221–224.

Kaupmann, K., Huggel, K., Heid, J. (1997). Expression cloning of GABA(B) receptors uncovers similarity to metabotropic glutamate receptors. *Nature* **386**, 223–224; 239–246.

Lafora, G.R. (1911). Über das Vorkommen amyloider Körperchen im Innern der Ganglienzellen; zugleich ein Beitrag zum Studium der amyloiden Substanz im Nervensystem. *Virchows Arch Path Anat* **205**, 295–303.

Lafora, G.R. and Glueck, B. (1911). Contribution to the histopathology and pathogenesis of myoclonic epilepsy. *Bull Gov Hosp Insane* **3**, 96.

Lander, E. and Schork, N. (1994). Genetic dissection of complex traits. *Science* **265**, 2037–2048.

Lee, A.G., Delgado-Escueta, A.V., Maldonado, H.M., Swartz, B.E. and Walsh, G.O. (1987). Closed-circuit television videotaping and electroencephalography biotelemetry (video/EEG) in primary generalized epilepsies. In: Gumnit, R.J. (Ed.), *Advances in Neurology, Vol. 46, Intensive Neurodiagnostic Monitoring.* Raven Press, New York, pp. 27–68.

Lewis, T.B., Leach, R.J., Ward, K. *et al.* (1993). Genetic heterogeneity in benign familial neonatal convulsions: identification of a new locus on chromosome 8q. *Am J Hum Genet* **53**, 670–675.

Liu, A.W., Delgado-Escueta, A.V., Serratosa, J.M. *et al.* (1995). Juvenile myoclonic epilepsy locus in chromosome 6p21.2-p11: linkage to convulsions and EEG trait. *Am J Hum Genet* **57**, 368–381.

Liu, A.W., Delgado-Escueta, A.V., Gee, M.N. *et al.* (1996). Juvenile myoclonic epilepsy in chromosome 6p12-p11: locus heterogeneity and recombinations. *Am J Med Gen* **63**, 438–446.

Loiseau, P. (1964). Crises épileptique survenant au réveil et épilepsie du réveil. *Sud Méd Chirug* **99**, 11492–11502.

Loiseau, P., Pestre, M., Dartigues, J.F., Commenges, D., Barbeger-Gateau, C. and Cohadon, S. (1983). Long-term prognosis in two forms of childhood epilepsy: typical absence seizures and epilepsy with rolandic (centrotemporal) EEG foci. *Ann Neurol* **13**, 642–648.

Mai, R., Canevini, M.P., Pontrelli, V. *et al.* (1990). L'epilepsia mioclonica giovanile di Janz: analisi prospettica di un campione di 57 pazienti. *Boll Lega It Epil* **70/71**, 307–309.

Marescaux, C., Vergnes, M. and Depaulis, A. (1992). Genetic absence epilepsy in rats from Strasbourg: a review. *J Neural Transm* **35** (suppl). 37–70.

Metrakos, K. and Metrakos, J.D. (1961a). Genetics of convulsive disorders. II. Genetic and electroencephalographic studies in centrencephalic epilepsy. *Neurology* **11**, 464–483.

Metrakos, K. and Metrakos, J.D. (1961b). Is the centrencephalic EEG inherited as a dominant? *Electroencephalogr Clin Neurophysiol* **13**, 289.

Metrakos, J.D. and Metrakos, K. (1969). Genetic studies in clinical epilepsy. In: Jasper, H.H., Ward, A.A., Pope, A. (Eds), *Basic Mechanisms of the Epilepsies*. Little Brown, Boston, pp. 700–708.

Metrakos, J.D., Metrakos, K., Polizos, P. *et al.* (1966). Genetics and ontogenesis of the centrecephalic EEG. *Electroencephalogr Clin Neurophysiol* **22**, 404.

Minassian, B.A., Lee, J.R., Hherbrick, J.A. *et al.* (1998). Mutations in a gene encoding a novel protein tyrosine phosphatase cause progressive myoclonus epilepsy, Lafora type. *Nat Genet* in press.

Minassian, B.A., Sainz, J., Serratosa, J.M. *et al.* (1999). Genetic locus heterogeneity in Lafora's progressive myoclonus epilepsy. *Ann Neurol* **45**, 262–265.

Morita, R., Miyazaki, E., Fong, C.Y.G. *et al.* (1998). JH8, a gene highly homologous to the mouse jerky gene, maps to the region for childhood absence epilepsy on 8q24. *Biochem Biophys Res Commun* **248**, 307–314.

Morita, R., Miyazaki, E., Delgado-Escueta, A.V. and Yamakawa, K. (1999). Exclusion of JH8 gene as a candidate for childhood absence epilepsy mapped to 8q24. *J Epilepsy Res* submitted.

Obeid, T. and Panayiotopoulos, C.P. (1988). Juvenile myoclonic epilepsy: a study in Saudi Arabia. *Epilepsia* **29**, 280–282.

Obeid, T., El Rab, M.O.G., Daif, A.K. *et al.* (1994). Is HLA-DRW13 (W6) associated with juvenile myoclonic epilepsy in Arab patients? *Epilepsia* **35**, 319–321.

Oller-Daurella, L. and Sanchez, M.E. (1981). Evolucion de las ausencias tipicas. *Rev Neurol* **9**, 81–102.

Panayiotopoulos, C.P. (1994). The clinical spectrum of typical absence seizures and absence epilepsies: In: Malafosse, A., Genton, P., Hirsch, E., Marescaux, C., Broglin, D. and Bernasconi, R. (Eds.), *Idiopathic Generalized Epilepsies*. John Libbey, London, pp. 75–86.

Panayiotopoulos, C.P. and Obeid, T. (1989). Juvenile myoclonic epilepsy: an autosomal recessive disease. *Ann Neurol* **25**, 440–443.

Panayiotopoulos, C.P., Obeid, T. and Waheed, G. (1989). Differentiation of typical absence seizures in epileptic syndromes. A video EEG study of 224 seizures in 20 patients. *Brain* **112**, 1039–1056.

Radovici, A., Misirliou, V. and Gluckman, M. (1932). Épilepsie reflexe provoquée par éxitation des rayons solaires. *Rev Neurol* **57**, 1305–1308.

Risch, N. (1991). A note on multiple testing procedures in linkage analysis. *Am J Hum Genet* **48**, 1058–1064.

Roger, J., Bureau, M., Dravet, Ch., Dreifuss, F.E., Perret, A. and Wolf, P. (1992). *Epileptic Syndromes in Infancy, Childhood and Adolescence*, second edition. John Libbey, London.

Sainz, J., Minassian, B.A., Serratosa, J.M. *et al.* (1997). Lafora's progressive myoclonus epilepsy: narrowing the 6q24 locus by recombinations and homozygosities. *Am J Hum Genet* **61**, 1205–1209.

Sander, T., Bockenkamp, B., Hildmann, T. *et al.* (1997a). Refined mapping of the epilepsy susceptibility locus EJM1 on chromosome 6. *Neurology* **49**, 842–847.

Sander, T., Kretz, R., Williamson, M.P. *et al.* (1997b). Linkage analysis between idiopathic generalized epilepsies and the GABA(A) receptor alpha5, beta 3 and gamma3 subunit gene cluster on chromosome 15. *Acta Neurol Scand* **96**, 1–7.

Sanguinetti, M.C., Curran, M.E., Spector, P.S. and Keating, M.T. (1996). Spectrum of HERG K+ channel dysfunction in an inherited cardiac arrhythmia. *Proc Natl Acad Sci U S A* **93**, 2208–2212.

Serratosa, J.M., Delgado-Escueta, A.V., Posada, I. *et al.* (1995). The gene for progressive myoclonus epilepsy of the Lafora type maps to chromosome 6q. *Hum Mol Genet* **4**, 1657–1663.

Serratosa, J.M., Delgado-Escueta, A.V., Medina, M.T. *et al.* (1996). Juvenile myoclonic epilepsy: D6S313 and D6S258 flank a 40 cM JME region. *Ann Neurol* **39**, 58–66.

Serratosa, J.M., Gómez-Garre, P., Gallardo, M.E. *et al.* (1999). A novel protein tyrosine phosphatase gene is mutated in progressive myoclonus epilepsy of the Lafora type (EPM2). *Hum Mol Genet* **8**, 345–352.

Singh, N.A., Charlier, C., Stauffer, D. *et al.* (1998). A novel potassium channel gene, KCNQ2, is mutated in an inherited epilepsy of newborns. *Nat Genet* **18**, 25–29.

Snead, O.C. (1994). Pathophysiological mechanisms of experimental generalized absence seizures in rats. In: Malafosse, A., Genton, P., Hirsch, E., Marescaux, C., Broglin, D., Bernasconi, R. (Eds), *Idiopathic Generalized Epilepsies: Clinical, Experimental, and Genetic Aspects*. John Libbey, London, pp. 133–150.

Toth, M., Grimsby, J., Buzsaki, G. and Donovan, G.P. (1995). Inactivation of a novel gene related to CENP-B is associated with neuronal hyperexcitability and seizure in transgenic mice. *Nat Genet* **11**, 71–75.

Wallace, R.H., Berkovic, S.F., Howell, R.A., Sutherland, G.R. and Mulley, J.C. (1996). Suggestions of a major gene for familial febrile convulsions mapping to 8q13-21. *J Med Genet* **33**, 308–312.

Weeks, D.E. and Lange, K. (1988). The affected pedigree member method of linkage analysis. *Am J Hum Genet* **42**, 315–326.

Weissbecker, K., Durner, M., Janz, D., Scaramelli, S., Sparkes, R.S., Spence, M.A. (1991). Confirmation of linkage between a juvenile myoclonic epilepsy-locus and the JLA-region of chromosome 6. *Am J Med Genet* **38**, 32–36.

Westling, B.W.H. (1997). A cluster of markers on chromosome 1 shows evidence for linkage to juvenile myoclonic epilepsy with absence in a large Mexican family [Thesis]. Louisiana State University.

Westling, B., Weissbecker, K., Serratosa, J.M. *et al.* (1996). Evidence for linkage of juvenile myoclonic epilepsy with absence to chromosome 1p. *Am J Hum Genet* **59**(S4), A1392.

Zara, F., Bianchi, A., Avanzini, G. *et al.* (1995). Mapping of genes predisposing to idiopathic generalized epilepsy. *Hum Mol Genet* **4**, 1201–1207.

Zara, F., Labuda, M., Bianchi, A., Garofalo, P.G., Durisotti, C. and Pandolfo, M. (1997). Evidence for a locus predisposing to idiopathic generalized epilepsies and spike-wave EEG on chromosome 3p14.2-p12.1. *Am J Hum Genet* **61**(S4), A43.

Zeng, Z., Kyaq, H., Gakenhimer, K.R. *et al.* (1997). Cloning, mapping, and tissue distribution of a human homologue of the mouse jerky gene produce. *Biochem Biophys Res Commun* **236**, 389–395.

Juvenile Myoclonic Epilepsy: The Janz Syndrome
Edited by Bettina Schmitz and Thomas Sander
© 2000 Wrightson Biomedical Publishing Ltd

15

Progress in Mapping the Gene for Juvenile Myoclonic Epilepsy (EJM1) within the Chromosomal Region 6p21.3

THOMAS SANDER,[a] BIRGIT BOCKENKAMP,[b] ANDREAS ZIEGLER[b] and DIETER JANZ,[a]

[a]*Epilepsy Genetics Group,* [b]*Department of Neurology and Institute for Immunogenetics, Charité Medical Faculty, Virchow Campus, Humboldt University of Berlin, Berlin, Germany*

INTRODUCTION

Juvenile myoclonic epilepsy (JME) is a common subtype of idiopathic generalized epilepsy (IGE), accounting for approximately 7% of all epilepsies (Janz, 1989, 1997). Its clinical features are characterized by bilateral myoclonic jerks, predominantly of arms and shoulders, without loss of consciousness. Myoclonic seizures occur shortly after awakening and start in adolescence. Absence seizures precede myoclonic jerks in about 30% of JME patients. In addition, generalized tonic-clonic seizures (GTCS), predominantly after awakening, occur in about 95% of JME patients. Approximately 5% of first-degree relatives of probands with JME will have epilepsy, of whom 30% will have JME and 30% will have an absence epilepsy (Beck-Mannagetta and Janz, 1991; Janz, 1997). Furthermore, paroxysmal generalized electroencephalographic (EEG) discharges, which indicate a bilateral synchronous neuronal hyperexcitability, are observed in up to 10% of otherwise healthy family members (Metrakos and Metrakos, 1961; Pedley, 1991). The remarkable phenotypic overlap of JME, absence epilepsies and the epilepsies with GTCS on awakening suggests that a shared genetic predisposition underlies the complex inheritance of this IGE spectrum (Berkovic *et al.*, 1987; Beck-Mannagetta and Janz, 1991; Janz *et al.*, 1992; Janz, 1997). Although genetic factors seem to be decisive in the aetiology of JME, the segregation of the epilepsy trait in families of JME probands indicates that several genetic factors contribute to its genetic susceptibility (Greenberg *et al.*, 1992; for review see: Sander, 1996).

Positional cloning is a step-wise procedure aiming for: (1) the mapping of a disease locus to a particular chromosomal region; (2) the identification and cloning of the responsible gene; (3) the detection of the trait-causing mutations; and (4) the elucidation of how the resulting alterations to the protein product causes disease. Linkage mapping of susceptibility loci is based on the tendency of genes to be inherited together in case of physical proximity on a chromosome (Lander and Schork, 1994). Susceptibility loci for JME can be mapped to chromosomal segments in family studies by demonstrating that the putative disease allele is inherited together with alleles of a polymorphic marker whose genomic map position is known. A rapidly increasing number of highly polymorphic markers facilitates linkage mapping. Once an IGE susceptibility locus has been assigned to a chromosomal segment, the current linkage map is reviewed to find potential candidate genes that can be included in further search procedures (e.g. mutational scanning techniques).

Two lines of evidence suggest that a susceptibility gene in the region of the human major histocompatibility (HLA) complex on the short arm of chromosome 6 contributes to the pathogenesis of JME and associated IGE syndromes. First, a significant association of JME with the HLA-DR13 allele has been reported in three independent studies (Durner et al., 1992; Obeid et al., 1994; Greenberg et al., 1996). Secondly, linkage studies of families ascertained through patients with JME provided evidence that a susceptibility gene for IGE, designated EJM1, maps to the HLA region (Greenberg et al., 1988; Durner et al., 1991; Sander et al., 1995; 1997). In addition, evidence for linkage of HLA markers with IGEs with generalized tonic-clonic seizures on awakening has been reported in families without JME-affected members (Greenberg et al., 1995). The EJM1-related phenotypic spectrum includes IGE seizure types with an age of onset towards adolescence, comprising JME, idiopathic absence epilepsies, and epilepsies with generalized tonic-clonic seizures on awakening (Sander et al., 1995). However, further studies have demonstrated that some families of JME patients do not show linkage to HLA (Elmslie et al., 1996; Liu et al., 1996). So far, linkage findings have been reported to the chromosomal regions 15q14 (Elmslie et al., 1997; Bate et al., this volume) and 6p11 (Liu et al., 1996; Serratosa et al., 1996), suggesting that genetic heterogeneity is an important issue in the complex genetic inheritance of JME. The present linkage study was designed to examine (1) the presence of the JME-related susceptibility locus (EJM1) in the chromosomal segment 6p21.3, and (2) to refine its map position in order to identify potential candidate genes in the region of interest.

METHODS

Families

The study protocol was approved by the Ethics Committee of the University Hospital Rudolf Virchow at the Free University of Berlin. Written informed consent was obtained from all participants. Twenty-nine German families with 277 members were selected through probands with JME. The diagnoses of epilepsies and epileptic syndromes were performed according to the proposal of the Commission on Classification and Terminology of the International League Against Epilepsy (1989).

DNA analyses

Genomic DNA was isolated from venous blood lymphocytes or lymphoblastoid cell lines (Miller et al., 1988). For linkage and haplotype analyses, 209 individuals were genotyped for 16 polymorphic markers from the chromosomal region 6p25 to 6q13 (Dib et al., 1996): telomere - 6p25 - D6S477 - (18.4 cM) - D6S289 - (5.0 cM) - D6S109 - (5.9 cM) - D6S299 - (3.0 cM) - D6S248 - (0.6 cM) - D6S273 - (0.3 cM) - HLA-DQA1/A2 - (3.0 cM) - D6S439 - (1.6 cM) - D6S291 - (5.5 cM) - D6S1019 - (5.4 cM) - D6S426 - (5.7 cM) - D6S271 - (7.7 cM) - D6S272 - (4.1 cM) - D6S295 - (1.8 cM) - D6S257 - (3.6 cM) - D6S254 - 6q13. Microsatellite genotyping was performed using standard polymerase chain reaction (PCR) protocols (Dib et al., 1996). Paternity of family members was confirmed by multi-locus genotyping.

Linkage analysis

Two-point linkage analyses were performed using the LINKAGE software package, version 5.1 (Lathrop and Lalouel, 1984). Multipoint linkage analysis was carried out using the program VITESSE (O'Connell and Weeks, 1995) for the following markers: D6S109, D6S248, HLA-DQA1/A2, D6S291 and D6S426. Marker distances were obtained from the current human genetic linkage map (Dib et al., 1996). Based on a previous exploration of the EJM1-related phenotypic spectrum, classification of affected subjects (n = 79) included 'idiopathic' generalized seizures (Sander et al., 1995). Family members exhibiting only other seizure types (e.g. febrile convulsions, symptomatic epilepsies) were classified as 'unaffected'. Clinically healthy individuals exhibiting generalized spike and wave discharges in their resting EEG (GSW-EEG) were designated as 'unknown' because of the high risk of genetic heterogeneity of this common and nonspecific subclinical trait marker. The analysis was carried out under an autosomal-dominant mode of inheritance with 70% penetrance, including a phenocopy rate of 1%, an age-of-onset correction and a frequency of the disease allele of 0.5%. Allele frequencies of the genetic markers were obtained from 112 clinically healthy founders of German families who participated in the present collaborative study on the genetics of IGE. The homogeneity of the linkage data was tested by the admixture test, implemented in the program HOMOG (Ott, 1983).

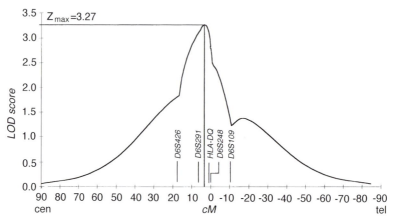

Figure 1. Multipoint linkage analysis of five microsatellite markers spanning a 15 cM region on either side of HLA with a susceptibility gene (EJM1) of 'idiopathic' generalized seizures in families of probands with juvenile myoclonic epilepsy. (Reproduced, with permission, from Sander *et al.*, 1997.)

RESULTS

Linkage analysis

Linkage analysis of 11 polymorphic markers from the chromosomal region 6p25-q13 revealed a peak LOD score of Z_{max} = 3.08 at the HLA-DQ locus, assuming genetic homogeneity and an autosomal dominant mode of inheritance with 70% penetrance. Multipoint analysis showed a peak Z_{max} = 3.27 at a map position about 3.3 cM centromeric to the HLA-DQ locus, assuming genetic homogeneity (Figure 1). The admixture test did not indicate evidence for heterogeneity among the families.

Haplotype analysis

Recombination events in family members affected by an IGE syndrome occurred in five families (Figure 2). Assuming genetic homogeneity, the chromosomal segment of overlap defines a candidate region for EJM1 centromeric to the HLA-DQ locus, spanning an interval of 10.1 cM flanked by the telomeric locus HLA-DQ and the centromeric locus D6S1019.

DISCUSSION

The present linkage results confirm previous linkage and association findings (for review see Sander, 1996), suggesting that a susceptibility locus (EJM1)

Chromosome 6

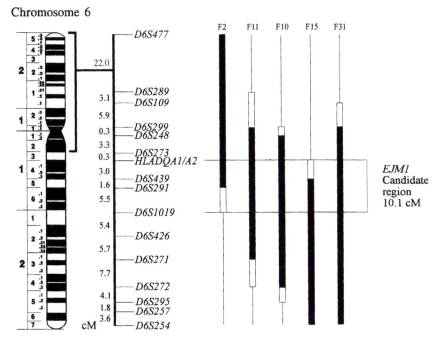

Figure 2. Map of 16 microsatellite loci in the chromosomal region 6p25-6q13 and recombination events in five families of JME patients. Dark bars indicate chromosomal segments that co-segregate with the EJM1 locus. The open bars represent the regions where recombinations occurred. The lines define chromosomal regions for which evidence against linkage has been obtained. Both the dark and shaded bars identify a candidate region for EJM1 in each family and the common segment of overlap. (Reproduced, with permission, from Sander *et al.*, 1997.)

for 'idiopathic' generalized seizures maps close to the HLA region on the chromosomal segment 6p21.3 in the majority of German families of JME patients. So far, significant evidence for two other susceptibility loci for JME has been reported. One susceptibility locus for JME has been mapped to the chromosomal region 6p11 in JME families lacking pyknoleptic absences (Liu *et al.*, 1996; Serratosa *et al.*, 1996). The other major locus for JME has been localized in the chromosomal region 15q14 (Elmslie *et al.*, 1997; Bate *et al.*, this volume) that harbours the gene encoding the α7 subunit of the neuronal nicotinic acetylcholine receptor (CHNRA7) (Freedman *et al.*, 1997). Taken together, the significant evidence for three different susceptibility loci for JME-related IGE syndromes indicates that genetic heterogeneity is an important factor in the complex genetic inheritance of JME. Accordingly, failure to replicate a linkage claim in oligogenic traits does not necessarily disprove initial linkage findings (Suarez *et al.*, 1994; Lernmark and Ott, 1998). Some susceptibility alleles will by chance be most prevalent in a given dataset, and those few target genes are unlikely to be prevalent in a similar proportion in a replication set.

The present haplotype analyses refine the candidate region of EJM1 to a 10 cM segment flanked by the loci HLA-DQ and D6S1019 (Sander *et al.*, 1997). However, it should be kept in mind that this refined candidate region is valid under the assumption of genetic homogeneity only. Recently, the authors have mapped the gene encoding the $GABA_B$ receptor ($GABA_BR1$) close to the HLA-F locus (Peters *et al.*, 1998). Accumulating evidence strengthens the role of $GABA_B$ receptors as important mediators of excitability mechanisms that generate paroxysmal epileptiform burst firing in neurons and aberrant synchronization in thalamocortical networks models (for review, see Caddick and Hosford, 1996). The functional properties of the $GABA_B$ receptor and its localization to the candidate region of the EJM1 locus on the chromosomal segment 6p21.3 emphasize the $GABA_BR1$ gene as a high-ranking candidate gene for the EJM1 gene. The authors have recently identified three exonic $GABA_BR1$ gene variants by single-strand conformation analysis in 18 unrelated German JME patients (Peters *et al.*, 1998) who were derived from families with positive evidence for linkage to the HLA-DQ locus (cumulative LOD score of $Z = 3.17$, assuming an autosomal-dominant inheritance with 70% penetrance) (Sander *et al.*, 1997). However, no evidence was found for an allelic association of any of these exonic $GABA_BR1$ variants with either JME or idiopathic absence epilepsies (Sander *et al.*, 1999). Thus, we failed to reveal evidence that genetic variation of the $GABA_BR1$ gene confers susceptibility to the pathogenesis of JME. Nonetheless, it is premature to exclude the $GABA_BR1$ gene as a candidate gene for JME. We are currently in the process of screening the promoter region of the human $GABA_BR1$ gene to identify regulatory elements for gene transcription.

In summary, the present linkage results strengthen evidence for a JME locus in the chromosomal region 6p21.3 and refine a tentative candidate region of 10 cM centromeric to the HLA-DQ locus. Evidence for two other major loci for JME in the chromosomal regions 6p11 and 15q14 indicates that more than one genetic factor is involved in the complex genetic inheritance of this disease, and that genetic heterogeneity plays an important role. Collaborative studies and a whole genome scan will be necessary to achieve sufficient statistical power to unravel the complex and heterogeneous genetic factors contributing to the genetic variance of JME.

ACKNOWLEDGEMENT

This chapter is dedicated to Dr Gertrud Beck-Mannagetta, who died in 1996, aged 47. It is unbelievable for all of us that someone so full of enthusiasm, ever-growing intellectual potential and so many human qualities died so prematurely.

This work was supported by the Deutsche Forschungsgemeinschaft (Be 1517/1-3; Sa 434/2-2, Ep 2/8-1), the European Union (GENE-CT93-0075), and the Stiftung Michael.

REFERENCES

Beck-Mannagetta, G. and Janz, D. (1991). Syndrome-related genetics in generalized epilepsy. *Epilepsy Res* **32** (suppl 4), 105–111.

Berkovic, S.F., Andermann, F., Andermann, E. and Gloor, P. (1987). Concepts of absence epilepsies: discrete syndromes or biological continuum? *Neurology* **37**, 993–1000.

Caddick, S.J. and Hosford, D.A. (1996). The role of $GABA_B$ mechanisms in animal models of absence seizures. *Mol Neurobiol* **13**, 23–32.

Commission on Classification and Terminology of the International League Against Epilepsy (1989). Proposal for revised classification of epilepsies and epileptic syndromes. *Epilepsia* **30**, 389–399.

Dib, C., Faure, S., Fizames, C. *et al.* (1996). The Genethon human genetic linkage map. *Nature* **380** (suppl), A95.

Durner, M., Sander, T., Greenberg, D.A., Johnson, K., Beck-Mannagetta, G. and Janz, D. (1991). Localization of idiopathic generalized epilepsies on chromosome 6p in families ascertained through juvenile myoclonic epilepsy patients. *Neurology* **41**, 1651–1655.

Durner, M., Janz, D., Zingsem, J. and Greenberg, D.A. (1992). Possible association of juvenile myoclonic epilepsy with HLA-DRw6. *Epilepsia* **33**, 814–816.

Elmslie, F.V., Williamson, M.P., Rees, M. *et al.* (1996). Linkage analysis in juvenile myoclonic epilepsy and microsatellite loci spanning 61 cM of human chromosome 6p in 19 nuclear pedigrees provides no evidence for a susceptibility locus in this region. *Am J Hum Genet* **59**, 653–663.

Elmslie, F.V., Rees, M., Williamson, M.P. *et al.* (1997). Genetic mapping of a major susceptibility locus for juvenile myoclonic epilepsy on chromosome 15q. *Hum Mol Genet* **6**, 1329–1334.

Freedman, R., Coon, H., Myles-Worsely, M. *et al.* (1997). Linkage of a neurophysiological deficit in schizophrenia to a chromosome 15 locus. *Proc Natl Acad Sci USA* **94**, 587–592.

Greenberg, D.A., Delgado-Escueta, A.V., Widelitz, H. *et al.* (1988). Juvenile myoclonic epilepsy (JME) may be linked to the Bf and HLA loci on chromosome 6. *Am J Med Genet* **31**, 185–192.

Greenberg, D.A., Durner, M. and Delgado-Escueta, A.V. (1992). Evidence for multiple gene loci in the expression of the common generalized epilepsies. *Neurology* **42** (suppl 5), 56–62.

Greenberg, D.A., Durner, M., Resor, S., Rosenbaum, D. and Shinnar, S. (1995). The genetics of idiopathic generalized epilepsies of adolescent onset: differences between juvenile myoclonic epilepsy and epilepsy with random grand mal and with awakening grand mal. *Neurology* **45**, 942–946.

Greenberg, D.A., Durner, M., Shinnar, S. *et al.* (1996). Association of HLA class II alleles in patients with juvenile myoclonic epilepsy compared with patients with other forms of adolescent-onset generalized epilepsy. *Neurology* **47**, 750–756.

Janz, D. (1989). Juvenile myoclonic epilepsy. *Cleveland Clin J Med* **56** (suppl 1), 23–33.

Janz, D. (1997). The idiopathic generalized epilepsies of adolescence with childhood and juvenile onset. *Epilepsia* **38**, 4–11.

Janz, D., Beck-Mannagetta, G. and Sander, T. (1992). Do idiopathic generalized epilepsies share a common susceptibility gene? *Neurology* **42** (suppl 5), 48–55.

Lander, E.S. and Schork, N.J. (1994). Genetic dissection of complex traits. *Science* **265**, 2037–2048.

Lathrop, G.M. and Lalouel, J.M. (1984). Easy calculations of lod scores and genetic risks on small computers. *Am J Hum Genet* **36**, 460–465.

Lernmark, A. and Ott, J. (1998). Sometimes it's hot, sometimes it's not. *Nat Genet* **19**, 213–214.

Liu, A.W., Delgado-Escueta, A.V., Gee, M.N. *et al.* (1996). Juvenile myoclonic epilepsy in chromosome 6p12-p11: locus heterogeneity and recombinations. *Am J Med Genet* **63**, 438–446.

Metrakos, J.D. and Metrakos, K. (1961). Genetics of convulsive disorders. II. Genetics and electro-encephalographic studies in centrencephalic epilepsy. *Neurology* **11**, 474–483.

Miller, S.A., Dykes, D.D. and Plesky, H.F. (1988). A simple salting out procedure for extracting DNA from human nucleated cells. *Nucleic Acids Res* **16**, 1215.

Obeid, T., el Rab, M.O., Daif, A.K. *et al.* (1994). Is HLA-DRw13 (w6) associated with juvenile myoclonic epilepsy in Arab patients? *Epilepsia* **35**, 319–321.

O'Connell, J.R. and Weeks, D.E. (1995). The VITESSE algorithm for rapid exact multilocus linkage analysis via genotype set-recording and fuzzy inheritance. *Nat Genet* **11**, 402–408.

Ott, J. (1983). Linkage analysis and family classification under heterogeneity. *Ann Hum Genet* **47**, 311–320.

Pedley, T. (1991). The use and role of EEG in the genetic analysis of epilepsy. *Epilepsy Res* **32** (suppl 4), 31–44.

Peters, C., Kämmer, G., Volz, A. *et al.* (1998). Precise mapping and genomic structure of the human $GABA_B R1$ receptor gene: no evidence of major involvement in idiopathic generalized epilepsy. *Neurogenetics* **2**, 47–54.

Sander, T. (1996). The genetics of idiopathic generalized epilepsy: implications for the understanding of its aetiology. *Mol Med Today* **2**, 173–180.

Sander, T., Hildmann, T., Janz, D. *et al.* (1995). The phenotypic spectrum related to the human epilepsy susceptibility gene 'EJM1'. *Ann Neurol* **38**, 210–217.

Sander, T., Bockenkamp, B., Hildmann, T. *et al.* (1997). Refined mapping of the epilepsy susceptibility locus EJM1 on chromosome 6. *Neurology* **49**, 842–847.

Sander, T., Peters, C., Kämmer, G. *et al* (1999). Association analysis of exonic variants of the gene encoding the $GABA_B$ receptor and idiopathic generalized epilepsy. *Am J Med Genet* in press.

Serratosa, J.M., Delgado-Escueta, A.V., Medina, M.T., Zhang, Q., Iranmanesh, R. and Sparkes, R.S. (1996). Clinical and genetic analysis of a large pedigree with juvenile myoclonic epilepsy. *Ann Neurol* **39**, 187–195.

Suarez, B.K., Hampe, C.L. and Van Eerdewegh, P. (1994). Problems of replicating linkage claims in psychiatry. In: Gershon, E.S. and Cloninger, C.R. (Eds), *Genetic Approaches to Mental Disorders*. American Psychiatric Press, Washington, DC, pp 23–46.

Juvenile Myoclonic Epilepsy: The Janz Syndrome
Edited by Bettina Schmitz and Thomas Sander
© 2000 Wrightson Biomedical Publishing Ltd

16

The Major Susceptibility Locus for Juvenile Myoclonic Epilepsy on Chromosome 15q

LOUISE BATE, MAGALI WILLIAMSON and MARK GARDINER

Department of Paediatrics, University College London, London, UK

INTRODUCTION

The molecular genetic basis of the idiopathic epilepsies is gradually being elucidated. The genes mutated in three Mendelian idiopathic epilepsies have been identified. Mutations in the gene CHRNA4, encoding the α4 subunit of the neuronal nicotinic acetylcholine receptor (nAChR) have been found in families with autosomal-dominant nocturnal frontal lobe epilepsy (ADNFLE) (Steinlein *et al.*, 1995). More recently, mutations in the genes KCNQ2 and KCNQ3, encoding two voltage-gated potassium channels, were discovered in families with benign familial neonatal convulsions (BFNC) (Charlier *et al.*, 1998; Singh *et al.*, 1998). In the same year, a mutation in SCNIB, the gene encoding the β1 subunit of the voltage-gated sodium channel, was found in a large pedigree with generalized epilepsy with febrile seizures plus (GEFS+) (Wallace *et al.*, 1998). To date, however, the genes responsible for the idiopathic epilepsies that display a complex mode of inheritance, including juvenile myoclonic epilepsy (JME), have proved elusive.

In this chapter, the mapping of a major susceptibility locus for JME on chromosome 15q, and the mutational analysis of the candidate gene which lies in this region, CHRNA7, are considered. In addition, results of linkage analysis of a broader phenotype, defined as idiopathic generalized epilepsy (IGE), with marker loci on chromosome 15q14 are described.

NEURONAL NICOTINIC ACETYLCHOLINE RECEPTORS AND IDIOPATHIC EPILEPSIES

Following the identification of mutations in CHRNA4 in families with ADNFLE, the genes encoding subunits of the neuronal nAChRs emerged as candidate genes for the inherited idiopathic epilepsies.

Neuronal nAChRs are heteropentameric ligand-gated ion channels. They are composed of various combinations of α and β subunits. The commonest configuration is of two α and three β subunits (Figure 3(a)). The α7 subunit apparently cannot co-assemble with other subunits, and forms a homomeric receptor/channel when expressed in *Xenopus* oocytes (Couturier *et al.*, 1990). The nAChRs differ in their expression pattern throughout the brain, and are thought to play a modulatory role in neurotransmitter transmission.

Eight genes for human nAChR subunits have been mapped: CHRNB2 (1p211-q21), CHRNA2 (8p21), CHRNAB3 (8p11.22), CHRNA7 (15q14), CHRNA3, A5, B4 (15q24), CHRNA4 (20q13.3) (Anand and Lindstrom, 1992; Chini et al., 1994).

To test the hypothesis that genes encoding subunits of nAChRs represent candidate susceptibility loci for JME, chromosomal regions harbouring genes for the eight mapped brain-expressed nAChR subunits were tested for linkage to the JME trait in multiplex nuclear families.

FAMILY RESOURCE

Thirty-four families including two or more individuals with clinical JME, were ascertained as part of a long-term European collaborative effort including a Concerted Action on the Genetic Analysis of Epilepsy.

Criteria for diagnosis were based on those of the International League Against Epilepsy (ILAE): an onset, between the ages of seven and 26 years, of generalized seizures, which must include myoclonic seizures, and may include absence seizures and generalized tonic-clonic seizures. Inter-ictal EEG patterns in patients showed episodes of generalized spike and wave or polyspike and wave discharges, with normal background activity. Patients had no abnormalities on neurological or neuroradiological examination (Commission on Classification and Terminology of the ILAE, 1989; Janz, 1985). Those with other epilepsy phenotypes, such as febrile convulsions or a single seizure, were classified as unknown. These thirty-four pedigrees contained 165 individuals of whom 73 were classified as affected, and five as unknown. All family members were aged 13 or over at the time of the last assessment.

METHODS

Genomic DNA was extracted from lymphocytes using standard methodology. Marker typing was carried out using fluorescence-based semi-automated methodology on an ABI 373 DNA sequencer (Perkin-Elmer, Foster City, CA, USA). The GAS package (version 2)© Alan Young 1993–1998, was used to convert absolute allele sizes to numbered alleles. Allele frequencies were estimated from the sample.

An initial screen with 22 polymorphic microsatellite markers spanning the chromosomal regions to which nAChR subunits map yielded negative LOD scores in all regions except the CHRNA7 region on chromosome 15q14. Further investigation was undertaken with eight highly polymorphic loci in this region, and the results analysed using parametric and nonparametric linkage analysis, implemented using the GENEHUNTER program (Kruglyak *et al.*, 1996).

PARAMETRIC AND NONPARAMETRIC ANALYSIS

Linkage analysis of complex traits is fraught with difficulty. Parametric analysis requires assumptions to be made about mode of inheritance and disease penetrance. Conventional thresholds of significance may not apply to linkage data derived from testing multiple models of inheritance, phenotype or genome-wide sets of markers.

Nonparametric analytical methods have been designed to overcome the problems of multiple modelling, as they are based on the likelihood of affected family members sharing alleles identical by state (IBS) or by descent (IBD) more often than would be expected by chance. It has been suggested that this form of analysis is the method of choice for the genetic analysis of complex traits. Methods which utilize IBS information cannot extract all the inheritance information from a pedigree, unlike those which are IBD-based, such as GENEHUNTER (Kruglyak *et al.*, 1996).

The GENEHUNTER program evaluates the multipoint inheritance pattern in the pedigrees, and calculates a scoring function to measure whether affected individuals share alleles identical by descent more often than would be expected under random segregation. No prior inheritance parameters are defined, but the admixture test to detect locus heterogeneity cannot be applied. The statistic produced, the nonparametric linkage (NPL) score, is referred to as the Z_{all} when sharing in sets larger than sib pairs is considered. The significance of the NPL score (p) can be calculated exactly.

RESULTS

Multipoint parametric analysis was carried out assuming either autosomal-dominant or autosomal recessive inheritance with 50% penetrance, and allowing for locus heterogeneity. Three liability classes were specified to allow for age-dependent penetrance.

Significant evidence in favour of linkage with heterogeneity was obtained. Multipoint parametric linkage analysis gave a maximum LOD score of 4.42 at

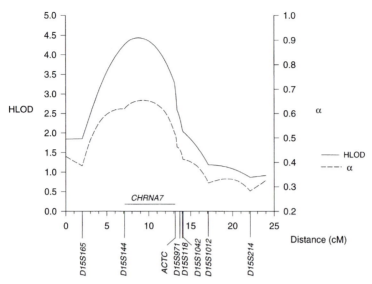

Figure 1. Graph of multipoint LOD score (HLOD) and corresponding values of α against genetic location on chromosome 15q. For clarity, the vertical axis denoting values of α has a baseline set at 0.2.

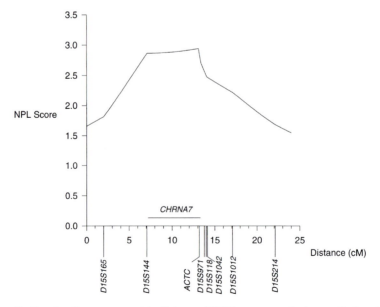

Figure 2. Graph of nonparametric linkage (NPL) score against genetic location on chromosome 15q.

a point 1.7 cM telomeric to D15S144 at $\alpha = 0.65$, assuming autosomal recessive inheritance (Figure 2). Non-parametric analysis of the data gave a maximum total score of $Z_{all} = 2.94$; $p = 0.00048$ at ACTC (Figure 3) (Elmslie *et al.*, 1997).

DISCUSSION

In this study a strong prior hypothesis, that genes encoding subunits of nAChRs are susceptibility loci for JME, was tested, in contrast to several recent studies in which random studies of the entire genome have been undertaken. A single narrow definition of the JME trait was used (according to criteria established by the ILAE). This, therefore, does not affect the threshold for statistical significance, and reduces the likelihood of introducing heterogeneity with a broad phenotype. Incorrect classification of nonpenetrant individuals as 'unaffected' may generate spurious exclusion data. In this study a low penetrance was assumed in order to reduce the likelihood of this occurring.

In the light of these considerations, the data presented therefore provide strong evidence in favour of a susceptibility locus for JME in this region that contributes to risk in a majority of the pedigrees analysed. Haplotype analysis shows the locus lies in a 15.1 cM region on chromosome 15q. The critical region encompasses CHRNA7, which has been mapped to the interval between D15S144 and ACTC using radiation hybrids, which corresponds to the region of peak LOD score.

The plausibility of CHRNA7 as a candidate for JME and mutational analysis of this gene is discussed below.

The α7 neuronal nicotinic acetylcholine receptor

CHRNA7 as a candidate gene for JME

Neuronal nAChRs are ligand-gated ion channels. Agonist binding to the extracellular domains of two α subunits of the receptor results in a conformational change, creating an open pore which allows the influx of cations, predominantly Ca^{2+} (Figures 3(a–d)). The neuronal receptors are composed of different combinations of α and β subunits to form oligomers, probably pentamers. Eight α (α2-9) and three β (β 2-4) subunit genes have been cloned (MeGehee and Role, 1995).

The α7-α9 nicotinic receptors form a distinct functional subclass of nAChRs based on their low affinity for nicotine, their high affinity for the snake toxin α-bungarotoxin (α-BGT) and their ability to form homo-oligomers *in vitro*. Of this class of receptors, only α7 is expressed throughout the mammalian brain. The α8 subunit has been found only in chicken

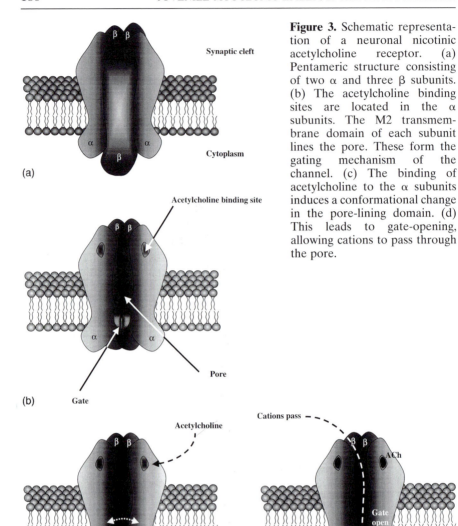

Figure 3. Schematic representation of a neuronal nicotinic acetylcholine receptor. (a) Pentameric structure consisting of two α and three β subunits. (b) The acetylcholine binding sites are located in the α subunits. The M2 transmembrane domain of each subunit lines the pore. These form the gating mechanism of the channel. (c) The binding of acetylcholine to the α subunits induces a conformational change in the pore-lining domain. (d) This leads to gate-opening, allowing cations to pass through the pore.

(Shoepfer *et al.*, 1990) and the α9 subunit has a very restricted expression in the pituitary and cochlear hair cells of the rat (Elgoyhen *et al.*, 1994). Unlike α1-6, the α7 subunits form functional homo-oligomeric channels when expressed in *Xenopus* oocytes (Couturier *et al.*, 1990). However, correct folding, assembly and subcellular localization of α7 transiently expressed in

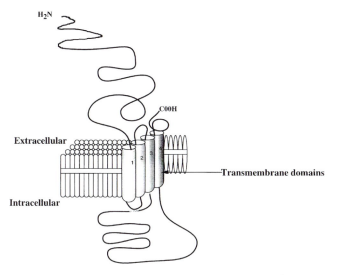

Figure 4. Schematic representation of a single nicotinic acetylcholine receptor subunit.

mammalian cell lines is dependent on host cell type (Cooper and Millar, 1997) and it is unclear whether α7 subunits form homo- or hetero-oligomeric receptors *in vivo*. The α7 and α8 subunits are thought to be the most primitive of AChR subunits (Le Novere and Changeux, 1995).

α7 subunits are structurally similar to the other nAChRs with an N-terminal extracellular domain involved in ligand binding, four hydrophobic transmembrane domains and a large cytoplasmic loop between transmembrane domains 3 and 4 (Figure 4). The CHRNA7 gene encodes a cDNA of 1.5 kb (Chini *et al.*, 1994) and is composed of 10 exons.

High levels of α7 gene expression have been shown in the nucleus reticularis of the thalamus (RTN), the lateral and medial geniculate bodies, the basilar pontine nucleus, the horizontal limb of the diagonal band of Broca, the nucleus basalis of Meynert and the inferior olivary nucleus in human post-mortem brain (Breese *et al.*, 1997). The RTN is thought to function as a pacemaker in corticothalamic innervation and has been implicated in the initiation of absence seizures in the rat (Snead, 1995). Expression of α7 mRNA is developmentally regulated in the rat brain; high levels are found into the first postnatal week followed by a decline into adulthood, although a widespread pattern of expression is maintained in the adult (Broide *et al.*, 1995).

Neuronal nAChRs are thought to be predominantly presynaptic and may have a role in modulating neurotransmitter release. Nicotine has been shown to stimulate the release of glutamate in an α-bungarotoxin (α-BGT)-blockable manner in rat hippocampal slice preparations (Gray *et al.*, 1996).

α7 receptors are thought to account for most of the α-BGT binding sites in the brain, as demonstrated in the CHRNA7 knock-out mouse in which high affinity α-BGT binding sites are absent. Increased concentrations of α-BGT binding sites have been found in mouse strains with an increased sensitivity to nicotine-induced seizures (Miner, 1986).

CHRNA7 is therefore a good candidate gene for JME due to its modulatory role in synaptic transmission in the CNS, its distribution in the brain and its association with nicotine-induced seizures in mice, as well as its chromosomal location.

Identification of a *CHRNA7*-related gene adjacent to *CHRNA7*

In order to determine whether mutations in CHRNA7 underlie the JME trait, reverse transcriptase-polymerase chain reaction experiments (RTPCR) were initially performed on RNA extracted from lymphoblastoid cell lines of JME probands. Amplification of exons 6–8 followed by direct sequencing identified a 2 base pair deletion of nucleotides 428-9 in exon 6, which would be predicted to result in a shift in the translational reading frame and premature termination of translation 40 amino acids downstream. This 2 base pair deletion was subsequently found in approximately 60% of controls at the genomic level, always in an apparently heterozygous state, demonstrating that this was not the disease-causing mutation, in spite of the expected severe consequences on the protein.

Additional evidence, including the coexistence of three alleles of an intragenic polymorphism in some individuals, led us to conclude that there was an additional locus with high homology to CHRNA7, with the 2 base pair deletion in the exon 6 equivalent of the CHRNA7-related gene. Somatic cell hybrid PCR and fluorescence *in situ* hybridization (FISH) results have shown that the α7 gene and the α7-related gene are adjacent and in close proximity on chromosome 15q14. Isolation of P1 and PAC clones of both genes has allowed the two genes to be sequenced and characterized independently.

The CHRNA7-related gene has an almost identical coding sequence to CHRNA7 from exons 5 to 10 of CHRNA7 with the same splice sites (Figure 5). The only potential protein-changing difference between the two genes in this region is the 2 base pair deletion in the exon 6 equivalent of the CHRNA7-related gene mentioned previously. This region of homology between the two genes includes the coding sequence for part of the N-terminal extracellular domain, the four transmembrane domains and the cytoplasmic loop. The 5' sequence of the CHRNA7-related gene has been determined by 5' RACE using a primer to CHRNA7 exon 5. This region is unique to the CHRNA7-related gene and has no homology to exons 1-4 of CHRNA7.

The high-sequence homology between the last three-quarters of the two genes suggests that the CHRNA7-related gene may have arisen from a partial

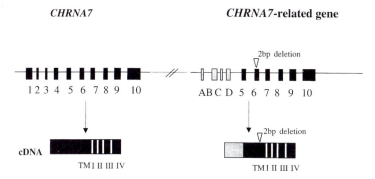

Figure 5. Diagram of the genomic structure of CHRNA7 and the CHRNA7-related gene.

duplication of CHRNA7. The CHRNA7-related gene is expressed *in vivo*; however, its function is unknown.

Mutational analysis of CHRNA7 and the related gene

Both genes are now being investigated as candidate genes for JME. The presence of two adjacent loci of high homology can frequently be the cause of large gene rearrangements such as deletions and gene conversion, as seen in spinal muscular atrophy and in steroid 21 hydroxylase deficiency (Lefebvre *et al.*, 1995; Tusie-Luna and White, 1995). The presence of such rearrangements is being investigated by Southern blotting and pulse field gel electrophoresis in DNA from JME probands.

Exons 1–4, which are unique to CHRNA7, are being screened for mutations by direct sequencing. Mutation analysis of exons 5–10 is more problematic, however. As the two genes are almost identical in this region, PCR amplification of any of the exons will generate amplified products from both genes. A heterozygous mutation in one gene would be represented by one in four of the amplified products, and so would be effectively masked by the control sequence.

To overcome these difficulties exons 5–10 are being screened for mutations by single-stranded conformation polymorphism (SSCP) analysis. This technique involves the denaturation of amplified products to make them single-stranded. The single strands are allowed to fold into sequence-specific conformations and are then separated on non-denaturing polyacrylamide gels. A single nucleotide change will result in the formation of a different conformation, which will have an altered mobility through the gel. Mutations in either gene would be detected using this technique. Any amplified products showing SSCP mobility shifts will be subcloned and individual clones sequenced. The functional significance of any amino acid sequence changes identified could then be assayed by *in vitro* expression of the mutations.

LINKAGE ANALYSIS OF IGE AND MARKER LOCI ON CHROMOSOME 15q14

Idiopathic generalized epilepsies

The IGEs are a group of epilepsies in which all seizures are generalized from onset, with a generalized bilateral synchronous, symmetrical discharge pattern on ictal EEG. Interictal EEG patterns in these patients may be normal, or show generalized spike, polyspike, spike and wave or polyspike and wave > 3 Hz against normal background activity. Patients have no abnormalities on neurological or neuroradiological examination (Commission on Classification and Terminology of the ILAE, 1989). Active IGE accounts for 90% of all generalized epilepsies (Hauser *et al.*, 1991).

This common group of epilepsies includes JME, juvenile absence epilepsy (JAE), childhood absence epilepsy (CAE) and epilepsy with generalized tonic-clonic seizures on awakening.

These epilepsies display a complex pattern of inheritance. Relatives of probands with IGE have a 5–8% risk of developing epilepsy (Janz *et al.*, 1989). Frequently, two or more different IGE phenotypes are found within a single pedigree, which suggests that there may be susceptibility loci that are common to all IGEs.

The aim of this study was to investigate whether this major susceptibility locus for JME contributes to genetic susceptibility in a broader phenotype, defined as IGE.

Family resource

Twelve pedigrees with a proband with JME and at least one first-degree relative with IGE were analysed. Families were ascertained as part of a long-term European collaborative effort, including a Concerted Action on the Genetic Analysis of Epilepsy (Figure 6).

Individuals were classified as affected if they had a clinical IGE using diagnostic criteria based on the ILAE classification of epilepsies and epileptic syndromes (Commission on Classification and Terminology of the ILAE, 1989). Individuals with other seizure disorders, febrile convulsions or a single seizure were classified as unknown.

These 12 pedigrees contained 92 individuals (82 genotyped) of whom 38 were classified as affected (35 genotyped) and three as unknown (two genotyped). All family members were aged eight or over at the time of the last assessment.

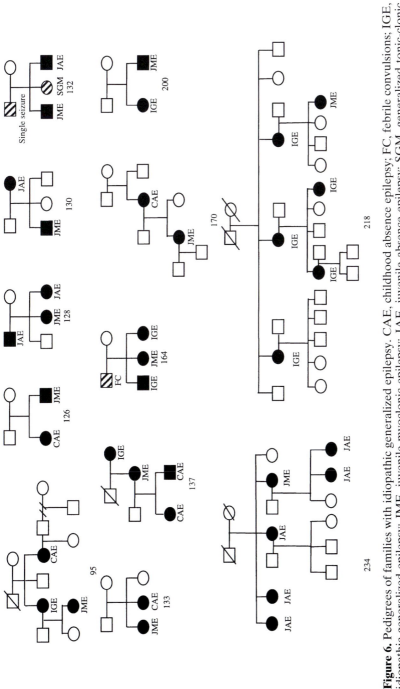

Figure 6. Pedigrees of families with idiopathic generalized epilepsy. CAE, childhood absence epilepsy; IGE, idiopathic generalized epilepsy; JME, juvenile myoclonic epilepsy; JAE, juvenile absence epilepsy; SGM, generalized tonic-clonic seizures during sleep. □, unaffected male; ○, unaffected female; ▨, unknown affective status; ■, affected male; ●, affected female; ⊘ ⌀, deceased individual.

Methods

Genomic DNA was extracted from lymphocytes using standard methodology. Individuals were typed with a set of four marker loci encompassing CHRNA7 on chromosome 15q14. Loci investigated were D15S144, ACTC, D15S971, and D15S118. Marker typing was carried out using fluorescence-based semi-automated methodology on an ABI 373 DNA sequencer. GAS (version 2) created by Alan Young was used to convert absolute allele sizes to numbered alleles. Allele frequencies were estimated from the sample. Parametric and nonparametric analysis of the data was carried out using the GENEHUNTER program (Kruglyak *et al.*, 1996). Multipoint parametric analysis was carried out assuming either autosomal dominant or autosomal recessive inheritance with 50% penetrance, and allowing for locus hetero-geneity. Three liability classes were specified to allow for age-dependent penetrance.

Results

No positive LOD scores were obtained. Significant exclusion (LOD score < -2) was obtained under all models (Figures 7 and 8). Nonparametric analy-sis of the data gave a maximum total Z_{all} of -0.59851 (not significant).

Discussion

The IGEs display a complex pattern of inheritance. This implies that several loci contribute to the observed genetic susceptibility. There may be a common locus or group of loci, perhaps acting to determine the seizure threshold, with additional loci contributing further phenotypic specificity.

   The aim of this project was to investigate whether, in this patient popula-tion, the susceptibility locus for JME on chromosome 15q14 conferred a genetic susceptibility to all IGEs, or if it is a phenotype-specific locus. The merits and pitfalls of parametric and nonparametric methods of analysis have been discussed earlier in the chapter. Unfortunately, this cohort is too small to generate significant results if the data are analysed using nonparametric methods.

   For parametric analysis, a low penetrance was assumed in order to reduce the possibility of nonpenetrant individuals being classified as 'unaffected', giving false-negative results. No individual family in this resource is powerful enough to achieve significant exclusion. However, assuming genetic homogeneity, overwhelming evidence for exclusion has been demonstrated in all the models tested. This suggests that, in these families, the susceptibility locus for JME on chromosome 15q14 is not a major susceptibility locus for IGE.

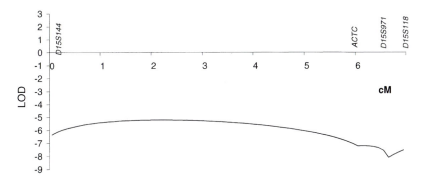

Figure 7. Graph of multipoint LOD score (autosomal recessive inheritance) against genetic location on chromosome 15q.

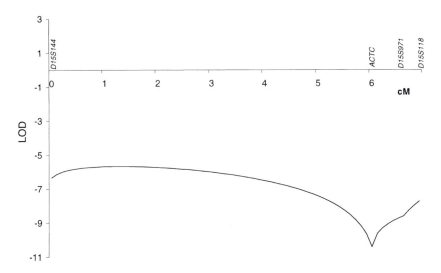

Figure 8. Graph of multipoint LOD score (autosomal dominant inheritance) against genetic location on chromosome 15q.

It may be argued that minor susceptibility loci for individual IGE phenotypes (e.g. JME, JAE, CAE) may be common to all subgroups, and determine the broad IGE disease phenotype, while major susceptibility loci for each IGE subgroup confer phenotype specificity. These phenotype-determining loci would therefore be expected to have less, if any, genetic influence when analysing the group of diseases as a whole. This could explain why the major susceptibility locus on chromosome 15q for JME does not appear to show linkage to the broader IGE phenotype.

CONCLUSIONS

A major susceptibility locus for JME on chromosome 15q has been mapped in 34 families in which two or more individuals have clinical JME. This region encompasses the gene for the α7 subunit of the neuronal nAChR, and mutational analysis of this gene has yielded interesting preliminary results. Linkage analysis of 12 families in which two or more first-degree relatives have an IGE, with marker loci on chromosome 15q14, gave overwhelming evidence for exclusion. This implies that the major susceptibility locus for JME on chromosome 15q does not contribute to genetic susceptibility in a broader phenotype, defined as IGE. This may be because the 15q locus acts to determine the specific JME phenotype, rather than having a broad role in conferring IGE susceptibility.

REFERENCES

Anand, R. and Lindstrom, J. (1992). Chromosomal localization of seven neuronal nicotinic acetylcholine receptor subunit genes in humans. *Genomics* **13**, 962–967.

Breese, C.R., Adams, C., Logel, J. *et al.* (1997). Comparison of the regional expression of nicotinic acetylcholine receptor alpha7 mRNA and [125I]-alpha-bungarotoxin binding in human postmortem brain. *J Comp Neurol* **387**, 385–398.

Broide, R., O'Connor, L., Smith, M., Smith, J. and Leslie, F. (1995). Developmental expression of alpha 7 neuronal nicotinic receptor messenger RNA in rat sensory cortex and thalamus. *Neuroscience* **67**, 83–94.

Charlier, C., Singh, N.A., Ryan, S.G. *et al.* (1998). A pore mutation in a novel KQT-like potassium channel gene in an idiopathic epilepsy family. *Nat Genet* **18**, 53–55.

Chini, B., Raimond, E., Elgoyhen, A.B., Moralli, D., Balzaretti, M. and Heinemann, S. (1994). Molecular cloning and chromosomal localisation of the human α7-nicotinic receptor subunit gene (CHRNA7). *Genomics* **19**, 37–381.

Commission on Classification and Terminology of the ILAE (1989). Proposal for revised classification of epilepsies and epilepsy syndromes. *Epilepsia* **30**, 389–399.

Cooper, S. and Millar, N. (1997). Host cell-specific folding and assembly of the neuronal nicotinic acetylcholine receptor alpha7 subunit. *J Neurochem* **68**, 2140–2151.

Couturier, S., Bertrand, D., Matter, J.M. *et al.* (1990). A neuronal nicotinic acetyl-choline receptor subunit (alpha 7) is developmentally regulated and forms a homo-oligomeric channel blocked by alpha-BTX. *Neuron* **5**, 847–856.

Elgoyhen, A.B., Johnson, D.S. Boulter, J., Vetter, D.E. and Heinemann, S. (1994). Alpha 9: an acetylcholine receptor with novel pharmacological properties expressed in rat cochlear hair cells. *Cell* **79**, 705–715.

Elmslie, F.V., Rees, M., Williamson, M.P. *et al.* (1997). Genetic mapping of a major susceptibility locus for juvenile myoclonic epilepsy on chromosome 15q. *Hum Mol Genet* **6**, 1329–1334.

Gray, R., Rajan, A., Radcliffe, K., Yakehiro, M. and Dani, J. (1996). Hippocampal synaptic transmission enhanced by low concentrations of nicotine. *Nature* **383**, 713–716.

Hauser, W., Annegers, J. and Kurland, L. (1991). Prevalence of epilepsy in Rochester, Minnesota: 1940–1980. *Epilepsia* **32**, 429–445.

Janz, D. (1985). Epilepsy with impulsive petit mal (juvenile myoclonic epilepsy). *Acta Neurol Scand* **72**, 449–459.

Janz, D., Durner, M. and Beck-Mannagetta, G. (1989). In: Beck-Mannagetta, G., Anderson, V., Doose, H. and Janz, D. (Eds), *Genetics of the Epilepsies*. Springer-Verlag, Berlin, pp. 43–52.

Kruglyak, L., Daly, M.J., Reeve-Daly, M.P. and Lander, E.S. (1996). Parametric and nonparametric linkage analysis: a unified multipoint approach. *Am J Hum Genet* **58**, 1347–1363.

Le Novere, N. and Changeux, J. (1995). Molecular evolution of the nicotinic acetyl-choline receptor: an example of multigene family in excitable cells. *J Mol Evol* **40**, 155-172.

Lefebvre, S., Burglen, L., Reboullet, S. *et al.* (1995). Identification and characterization of a spinal muscular atrophy-determining gene. *Cell* **80**, 155–165.

McGehee, D. and Role, L. (1995). Physiological diversity of nicotinic acetylcholine receptors expressed by vertebrate neurons. *Annu Rev Physiol* **57**, 521–546.

Miner, L.L., Marks, M.J. and Collins, A.C. (1986). Genetic analysis of nicotine-induced seizures and hippocampal nicotinic receptors in the mouse. *J Pharmacol Exp Ther* **239**, 853–860.

Orr-Urtreger, A., Goldner, F., Saeki, M. *et al.* (1997). Mice deficient in the alpha7 neuronal nicotinic acetylcholine receptor lack alpha-bungarotoxin binding sites and hippocampal fast nicotinic currents. *J Neurosci* **17**, 9165–9171.

Shoepfer, R., Conroy, W., Whiting, P., Gore, M. and Lindstrom, J. (1990). Brain alpha-bungarotoxin binding protein cDNAs and MAbs reveal subtypes of this branch of the ligand-gated ion channel gene superfamily. *Neuron* **5**, 35–48.

Singh, N.A., Charlier, C., Stauffer, D. *et al.* (1998). A novel potassium channel gene, *KCNQ2*, is mutated in an inherited epilepsy of newborns. *Nat Genet* **18**, 25–29.

Snead, O. (1995). Basic mechanisms of generalized absence seizures. *Ann Neurol* **37**, 146–157.

Steinlein, O.K., Mulley, J.C., Propping, P. *et al.* (1995). A missense mutation in the neuronal nicotinic acetylcholine receptor alpha 4 subunit is associated with autosomal dominant nocturnal frontal lobe epilepsy. *Nat Genet* **11**, 201–203.

Tusie-Luna, M. and White, P. (1995). Gene conversions and unequal crossovers between CYP21 (steroid 21-hydroxylase gene) and CYP21P involve different mechanisms. *Proc Natl Acad Sci U S A* **92**, 10796–10800.

Wallace, R.H., Wang, D.W., Singh, R. *et al.* (1998). Febrile seizures and generalised epilepsy associated with a mutation in the Na+ channel beta1 subunit gene SCNIB. *Nat Genet* **19**, 366–370.

Juvenile Myoclonic Epilepsy: The Janz Syndrome
Edited by Bettina Schmitz and Thomas Sander
© 2000 Wrightson Biomedical Publishing Ltd

17

Quo Vadis?

DIETER JANZ

Epilepsy Research Group, Charité Medical Faculty, Virchow Campus, Humboldt University, Berlin, Germany

I am sure the organizers did not think of me, but of the syndrome, when they asked me to spare some thoughts on this question at the end of the symposium. The question, therefore, should be, in fact, Quo vadis JME? If I am, however, identified with the syndrome to such an extent that I, in its place, have to speak about where it is going, then I must seriously question myself about how I feel.

Jackson was once asked whether he minded that the seizures he had classified as 'epileptiform' were now named after him, a proposal of Charcot's. To this Jackson replied with the lapidary statement, that he had to live with it. However, according to his own views, all types of seizures were Jacksonian. In fact, he meant to say, it is not the label that is important, but rather his view of inferring pathophysiological mechanisms from clinical observations. In a similar fashion, rather than insisting on my original descriptions of individual syndromes, such as pyknolepsy as a kind of 'petit-mal epilepsy' (Janz, 1955) and sleep epilepsy and awakening epilepsy (Janz, 1962) as different types of grand mal epilepsy, I would prefer to see my name in connection with a clinically differentiating nosological view on epilepsy, of which JME has indeed become an almost classical example.

As Peter Wolf mentioned earlier in this volume, JME could be viewed as a model for the descriptions of other epileptic syndromes. But JME is also evidence of the fact that, from a research point of view, the generalized epilepsies are as interesting as the focal epilepsies, and the idiopathic as stimulating as the symptomatic epilepsies. For a long time it seemed that in the field of epilepsy research all interests were absorbed in investigating those epilepsies for which there was a demonstrable, visible, localized and surgically removable cause. Thus, the impression was given that the generalists no longer waved their modest flag against the focalists. However, reviewing the results of this meeting, research interest in generalized epilepsies has been rejuvenated, as it has been shown that scientific criteria such as visualization, confirmation and a technical approach are also applicable in this field.

When, in conjunction with Meencke, the author postulated that the small neuronal abnormalities found in the brains of patients with idiopathic generalized epilepsy (Meencke and Janz, 1984, 1985) were due to early disturbances in brain maturation, we were told that 'idiopathic' is characterized by the fact that there are no morphological brain lesions to be found (Lyon and Gastaut, 1985). Morgenstern summarized these arguments splendidly by saying *daß nicht sein kann, was nicht sein darf* meaning that our description contradicted the generally accepted definition of idiopathic. Now, as shown in this volume by Woermann and Duncan and Koepp and Duncan (Chapters 8 and 9, this volume), one can detect with new imaging techniques structural as well as metabolic abnormalities in patients with JME. Once again one will hear that this type of epilepsy is symptomatic. However, it does not make sense to move the border between idiopathic and symptomatic as soon as new investigation techniques become available. Notwithstanding, these new insights force us to acknowledge that the idiopathic epilepsies not only have a correlate on the neurophysiological, or functional level, but also on the morphological and neurobiological level, which can now be investigated and detected *in vivo*. Both the morphological evidence described by Meencke (1983), plus earlier electrophysiological studies presented here by Avanzini *et al.* (Chapter 6, this volume) as well as the neuropsychological data presented by Trimble (Chapter 10, this volume), agree with the results of imaging techniques, pointing towards a frontal lobe dysfunction. Thus, JME proves to be clinically consistent and precise, and this makes JME prone to being a model for the investigation of other syndromes of idiopathic generalized epilepsies.

This raises then the question of the appropriate place for concentrated research into idiopathic generalized epilepsy. This is probably not the epilepsy centre interested in preoperative monitoring and surgical treatment, where one might also find these patients, but more accidentally because of being wrongly diagnosed. Patients with JME and with other variants of epilepsies on awakening are preferentially seen in neurological practices and specialized epilepsy clinics for outpatients of neurological departments, according to Loiseau *et al.* (1991) even more often in private practice than in general neurological outpatient departments.

Patients with idiopathic generalized epilepsies are obviously not an urgent problem from a general health point of view. They are easy to treat, if you provide the correct diagnosis and early treatment with the appropriate drug and the adequate handling of the psychopedagogical context. But they play a key role in the whole of epilepsy research. Whoever carries the genetic key to JME will be able to shed light onto other complex inherited types of epilepsy.

Is this where JME is going? No one will hesitate to postulate, especially under the impression of the work and the presentations of Delgado-Escueta *et al.* (Chapter 14, this volume), Durner *et al.* (1998), Gardiner (see Bate *et al.*, Chapter 16, this volume), Sander *et al.* (Chapter 15, this volume) and Greenberg *et al.* (1998) that the future lies in the field of molecular genetics. Now, only the positional cloning of the major loci and the systematic scanning of the whole genome need to be carried out in order to detect further susceptibility loci, to get a grip on the genetic defects and constellation of mutations. But this book shows that this is not going to happen quickly. Even Antonio Delgado-Escueta, who tried to encourage me in the summer 1990, when I was depressed about the fact that our LOD score had fallen again, told me, 'Don't worry, Dieter, we will find the gene in the autumn!' Now even he has become more conservative with prognoses of time. What is the reason for this?

Some presentations have indicated that we might have underestimated the syndrome. We regarded it as too simple. We have not considered the complexity of the simplicity (Janz and Sander, 1999), in terms of its syndrome-specific symptomatology as well as its place within the overall category of generalized epilepsies. We also lack a theoretical concept, which combines type of disease, symptomatology and course within one neurobiological context. My earlier hypothesis that all syndromes of generalized epilepsies should be considered as variants of paroxysmal dysfunctions in the ontogenetic development of static functions (Janz, 1998) has never been picked up by neurophysiologists and neurobiologists.

This critical reflection could, however, open up new perspectives through stronger emphasis on what we have learned in this volume, namely to consider carefully the conditions for triggering the jerks, these 'micro-situations' composed of varying levels of vigilance and behaviour, and also the jerks themselves, their dynamics, and distribution, both localized and regional. In particular, the practically exclusive distinction of photosensitivity and praxis sensitivity as demonstrated by Inoue and Kuboto (Chapter 7, this volume) is a new and hopeful acquisition. The notion of such symptomatologic and dynamic similarities and differences within an intra- and inter-family context could first of all help the geneticists to overcome the problem of heterogeneity with the task of defining subgroups which are as homogeneous as possible.

Such a differentiating view has often been criticized or ridiculed by the simplifiers of our guild as splitting. But I interpret splitting as refining the diagnosis, which is as important for genetic science as it is for therapy. Following the same principles, refining the details of individual patients' histories is equally beneficial for therapy, as it supports the patient's reflections about himself or herself and their coping with the conditions of the disease, and by this means, strengthens their self-control. If we use the newly gained insights illustrated here in such a way, then JME could become an exemplifying model of research as well as a paradigm for the therapy of idiopathic generalized epilepsies.

REFERENCES

Durner, M., Greenberg, D.A., Shinnar, S.S. *et al.* (1998). No evidence for linkage of juvenile myoclonic epilepsy to chromosome 15. *Epilepsia* **39** (suppl 6), 145.

Greenberg, D.A., Durner, M., Shinnar, S.S. *et al.* (1998). Linkage analysis on chromosome 6 shows evidence for heterogeneity within the JME syndrome. *Epilepsia* **39** (suppl 6), 144–145.

Janz, D. (1955). Die klinische Stellung der Pyknolepsie. *Dtsch Med Wochenschr* **80**, 1392–1400.

Janz D. (1962). The grand mal-epilepsies and the sleeping-waking cycle. *Epilepsia* **3**, 69–109.

Janz, D. (1998). *Die Epilepsien-Spezielle Pathologie und Therapie*, 2nd edn. Thieme, Stuttgart, pp. 159–161.

Janz, D. and Sander, T. (1999). Juvenile myoclonic epilepsy: the complexity of a simple syndrome. In: Kotagal, P. and Lüders, H.O. (Eds), *The Epilepsies: Etiologies and Prevention*. Academic Press, San Diego, CA, pp. 561–570.

Loiseau, P., Duché, B. and Loiseau, J. (1991). Classification of epilepsies and epileptic syndromes in two different samples of patients. *Epilepsia* **32**, 303–309.

Lyon, G. and Gastaut, H. (1985). Considerations on the significance attributed to unusual cerebral histological findings recently described in eight patients with primary generalized epilepsy. *Epilepsia* **26**, 365–367.

Meencke, H.J. (1983). The density of dystopic neurons in the white matter of the gyrus frontalis inferior in epilepsies. *J Neurol* **230**, 171–181.

Meencke, H.J. and Janz, D. (1984). Neuropathological findings in primary generalized epilepsy: A study of eight cases. *Epilepsia* **25**, 8–21.

Meencke, H.J. and Janz, D. (1985). The significance of microdysgenesia in primary generalized epilepsy: an answer to the consideration of Lyon and Gastaut. *Epilepsia* **26**, 368–371.

Morgenstern, C. (1978). *Galgenlieder etca.* Reclam, Stuttgart, p. 81.

Index

A

absence epilepsies
  classification 138, 139, 141
  frequency in first-degree relatives 138
  genetic linkage and 142
  see also childhood absence epilepsy
    (CAE); juvenile absence epilepsy
    (JAE)
absences
  in JME 13–14, 19, 48
    age at onset 16
    EEG 52, 53
    incidence/prevalence 19, 136–137
    pathophysiology and opioid release 93
acetazolamide 23
acetylcholine
  binding to receptor 186
  nicotinic receptor *see* nicotinic
    acetylcholine receptor
age of onset
  childhood absence epilepsy (CAE) 134, 135
  idiopathic generalized epilepsy (IGE) 134,
    135
  inheritance of susceptibility and 140
  JME 13, 15–16, 133
  juvenile absence epilepsy (JAE) 134, 135
  Lafora's progressive myoclonus epilepsy
    146
  Lennox–Gastaut syndrome 135
  myoclonic jerks 16
  praxis-induced seizures 75
alcohol consumption 17, 106, 112
alpha-fetoprotein 127
antiepileptic drugs, in JME 23–24
  aggravating effects 23–24
  behavioural changes after 106
  compliance 112
  discontinuation and seizure relapse 116–118
  favourable response, definition 111–112
  poor response 114–115
  relapse rate after discontinuation 111–120
  response 111, 112–115, 115–116
  seizure recurrence with 112–115
ascertainment bias 112, 118
auditory precipitation 115

Aufwach-epilepsy 103
autosomal-dominant nocturnal frontal lobe
  epilepsy (ADNFLE) 181
awakening, sudden
  forced normalization and 106, 107
  JME and 20, 105–106, 107
  myoclonic jerks 17, 18, 20, 73
awakening grand mal 26

B

baclofen 164–165
behavioural changes
  after anticonvulsants 106
  JME 102
behavioural disorders
  after maternal use of valproate 123
  in JME 20
benign familial neonatal convulsions (BFNC)
  161, 162, 181
benign grand mal 26
benign myoclonic epilepsy in infancy
  (BMEI) 26
benzodiazepines 97
Bewegungsmotiv 2
Blitz–Nick–Salaam seizures 135, 138
brain
  contours 84–85
  disorders, valproate use in pregnancy
    121–128
  see also entries beginning cerebral
α-bungarotoxin 185, 187

C

carbamazepine 24
CCTV-EEG 145, 149, 156
cDNA
  GABA-B receptors 165
  jerky gene 166
central benzodiazepine receptor (CBZR)
  93–97
  flumazenil binding as marker 94–95
cerebral blood flow, regional 92, 93
cerebral cortex
  functional disorganization 95
  structural changes 83–89

cerebral glucose metabolism, regional 92
childhood absence epilepsy (CAE) 25–26, 48
    age of onset 134, 135
    candidate genes 166
    clinical features 139
    gene loci 146, 147, 157–160
        CAE evolving to JME (chromosome 1p)
            146, 147, 154–156
        chromosome 8q24 146, 158, 159, 166
        chromosome 8q loci 161–162
        see also chromosome 8q24
    grey matter volume 85
    inheritance risk 133
    juvenile absence epilepsy vs 135–136
    overlap with other syndromes 136, 137,
        141
        JME 136, 141
    photosensitivity rate 48
    self-remitting subsyndrome 157
    subsyndromes 157, 159
childhood pyknoleptic absence epilepsy 157
CHRNA4 gene 181
CHRNA7 gene
    exons 187, 189
    expression, sites 187
    gene adjacent see CHRNA7-related gene
    as JME candidate gene 185–190
    mutational analysis 189–190
    structure 188, 189
CHRNA7-related gene 188–190
    mutational analysis 189–190
    structure 188, 189
chromosome 1p
    childhood absence epilepsy evolving to
        JME 146, 147, 154–156
    JME with pyknoleptic absences 154–156
    photogenic childhood absences with eyelid
        myoclonias 156–157
chromosome 2p 156–157
chromosome 6p 146, 177
    candidate gene for JME
        GABA-B receptor 164–165
        jerky gene 165–166
    classic JME 35, 146, 147, 149–150,
        150–154
    heterogeneity 149–150, 153–154, 164, 178
    initial proof 150
    linkage studies 151, 152
    multipoint analysis and recombinations
        151–153
    non-6p-linked families and 153–154
    gene number 163–164
    gene within/below HLA 163–164
    region 6p11 177, 178
    region 6p21.3, EJM1 gene locus 174–180
    region 6p25–6q13 177
chromosome 6q, mutation in Lafora's disease

148
chromosome 8p24, human jerky gene and 166
chromosome 8q
    loci for childhood absence epilepsy
        161–162
    region 8q13–21 162
chromosome 8q24 147
    childhood absence epilepsy locus 158, 159,
        160–162
        family study 160–162
        multiplex families 161–162
        recombination events and critical region
            161
chromosome 12p 156–157
chromosome 15q14 177, 178, 181
    CHRNA7 gene 185–190
    JME susceptibility locus 185–190, 192
chromosome 19q 156–157
chronosensitivity 20, 21, 27
circadian distribution of seizures 20, 21
classification of epilepsy 134
clinical features, of JME 5, 7, 13, 27, 59, 64,
    139
clinical genetics see genetics of epilepsy
clonazepam 114
clonic-tonic-clonic seizures 19
cognitive studies 104–105
commotions 6
compliance, drug 112
computed tomography (CT) 22
concordance, syndromic
    factors associated 139, 140
    rates, idiopathic generalized epilepsy
        subtypes 137, 140
congenital malformations, valproate use in
    pregnancy 121–128
consanguinity, Lafora's progressive
    myoclonus epilepsy 148
corticospinal system, activation in myoclonic
    jerks 69

D
definition, of JME 1–2, 11, 12–14, 33–34
diabetes mellitus 21
diagnosis, of JME 14, 28
    delays 17–18, 24
    EEG role 52–53
    features 27
    by referring physicians 17
    related epileptic syndromes 24–25
    see also misdiagnosis
diprenorphine 91, 93
DNA
    analyses in JME gene locus studies 175
    complementary see cDNA
drug-resistant JME 23, 115
duration of JME 13

E
EBN2 gene locus 161
EJM1 gene 142, 163
　candidate region by haplotype analysis 178
　HLA region and 163–164
　JME and absences linked 142
　mapping 173–180
　　chromosome 6p21.3 176–177
electroencephalography (EEG) 1, 59–61
　CCTV recorded 145, 149, 156
　idiopathic generalized epilepsy 12, 41, 45
electroencephalography (EEG), in JME 12,
　27, 34, 41–55
　with absences 52, 53
　alpha-EEG 51–52
　arousal-related changes and discharges
　　63–64, 70
　background activity 51–52
　diagnostic value 52–53
　eye closure effect 49–50, 50
　focal findings 50–51
　hyperventilation effect 46–47
　ictal discharges 46
　interictal discharges 42, 69
　misinterpretation 52, 53
　myoclonus relationship to discharges 61–63
　photosensitivity 47–50, 73
　polyspikes 12, 42, 44
　polyspike-waves 12, 27, 34, 41, 43–46, 63–64
　　amplitudes and frequency 45
　　ictal 46
　　interictal 42, 43
　　slow waves preceding 46
　praxis-induced seizures 78, 79
　sleep and sleep deprivation effect 47
　spikes and waves 12, 34, 41–43, 44
　spike-waves 70
　　thalamocortical system 92, 97
　voltage asymmetry 51
electromyography (EMG) 60
endozepines 97
epilepsy see individual types of epilepsy,
　features
epileptic syndromes, associated with JME
　24–25, 28
epileptology 33
European history, of JME 5–9
evolution of JME 22–23
eye closure, sensitivity 49–50, 50
eyelid myoclonia 26
　with absences see photogenic childhood
　　absence with eyelid myoclonia

F
familial myoclonus epilepsy 6
familial recurrence rate 131
　in first-degree relatives 138

families, large, use in gene locus studies 151,
　152, 162–163
family history, of JME 14–15, 75
11C-flumazenil 91, 93–94
　areas of increased binding 94, 95
　as marker of central benzodiazepine
　　receptor 94–95
focal epilepsy 21
　genetics 133
folic acid supplementation 126, 127
forced normalization 105–107, 107
　in awakening epilepsy 106, 107
formylated tetrahydrofolates 126
Friedmann syndrome 7
frontal lobe
　dysfunction 7, 20
　functional tests 104–105
　impairment in JME 105
　mesial 86, 87
frontal lobe epilepsy 105
　autosomal-dominant nocturnal (ADNFLE)
　　181

G
GABA 93–94, 95
　agonists 97
　receptors 164
GABA-A receptors 97, 165
GABA-B receptors 164–165, 178
　antagonists 165
　cDNAs 165
　$GABA_BR1$ gene variants 178
　gene as candidate gene for JME 164, 178
　HGABABR 165
gamma-aminobutyric acid (GABA) see GABA
gene(s)
　candidate
　　for childhood absence epilepsy
　　　164–166
　　CHRNA7 see CHRNA7 gene
　　for JME 164–166, 174–180, 199
　epilepsy syndromes 130
　in JME 145–171
　linkage studies see linkage analysis
　loci 34, 146
　　childhood absence epilepsy 157–160
　　classic JME 149, 150–154
　　heterogeneity in classic JME 34,
　　　149–150, 153–154, 164, 183
　　idiopathic generalized epilepsy 146, 147,
　　　174
　　Lafora's progressive myoclonus epilepsy
　　　146–149
　　pyknoleptic absences in JME 153–154
　　use of large families in studies 151, 152,
　　　162–163
　　see also specific chromosomes

mapping methods 174
translocation 34
GENEHUNTER program 183, 192
generalized epileptic activity, in JME 38–39
generalized tonic-clonic seizures (GTCS) 1,
    13–14
  age at onset 16
  characteristics 19
  myoclonic jerks preceding 19
  overlap with other syndromes 136, 137
  triggering factors 17
generalized tonic clonic seizures on
    awakening (GTCSA) 133, 136
  combination of syndromes with 136–137
  frequency in first-degree relatives 138
GENES international consortium 149, 157
Genetic Absence Epilepsy Rat from
    Strasbourg (GAERS) 69
genetic counselling 141
genetic linkage see linkage analysis
genetics of epilepsy 130–134
  evidence for role 131
  frequency in first-degree relatives 138
  of idiopathic generalized epilepsy subtypes
    129–144
  of JME 14–15, 34
  offspring risks 130–131, 132, 141
  sibling risks 131, 132, 133
genetic susceptibility 173
genetic variability 129
gestalt perception 1–3
grand mal (GM) seizure 1
  awakening 26
  benign 26
  pure awakening syndrome 147
grey matter volumes 85, 86

H
haplotype analysis, JME 176, 178
heterogeneity, definition 129
history, of JME 5
HLA-DQ 163, 164, 176, 178
HLA-DRw6 164
HLA-F 178
HLA loci
  chromosome 6p epilepsy gene relationship
    163–164, 173
  classic JME loci linked 150, 151, 173
homogeneous syndromes 34–35
hyperthyroidism 21
hyperventilation 46–47
hypothyroidism 21

I
idiopathic generalized epilepsy (IGE) 5, 6,
    7, 190, 198
  age of onset 134, 135

complex inheritance 192
  as continuum 134, 142
  definition 12
  EEG 12, 41, 45
  family pedigrees 190, 191
  genetic loci 146, 147, 174
  genetics of subtypes 129–144
    see also genetics of epilepsy
  grey matter volume 85
  JME related syndromes 26, 28
  linkage analysis of chromosome 15q14 loci
    190–194
  pathology 83–84
  positron emission tomography 91–99
  prevalence 14
  prognosis 137–138
  recurrence risk in offspring 141
  research 198
  subtypes 12, 134, 190
    combinations 136–137
    intrafamilial syndrome concordance
      137, 138, 139, 140
    intraindividual overlap 136, 137, 141
    overlap between 141
  terminology 198
impulsions 2, 6
impulsive petit mal 1, 2, 6–7, 33–34, 145
    see also juvenile myoclonic epilepsy (JME)
inheritance of epilepsy 129, 130–134
    see also genetics of epilepsy
intellectual ability, child after maternal use
    of valproate 123
intelligence quotients (IQs) 104–105
International Classification of Epilepsies and
    Related Syndromes 12, 33, 134
International League Against Epilepsy 2, 41,
    112
intrafamilial syndrome concordance 137,
    138, 139, 140

J
Jacksonian seizures 197
Janz, Dieter 1–3, 5, 7, 102, 107, 197–200
Janz epilepsy gene 146
Janz syndrome 1–3
  origin of name and early description 1–3,
    6, 7
    see also juvenile myoclonic epilepsy (JME)
jerk-locked averaging (JLA) 60, 61
jerks
  history and early description 1, 2, 6
    see also myoclonic jerks
jerky gene 165–166
  cDNA 166
juvenile absence epilepsy (JAE) 25–26, 48
  age of onset 134, 135
  childhood absence epilepsy vs 135–136

clinical features 139
grey matter volume 85
JME overlap 136, 141
overlap with other syndromes 136, 137, 141
photosensitivity rate 48
juvenile myoclonic epilepsy (JME)
as complex syndrome xi, 33–39, 199
definition 1–2, 11, 12–14, 33–34
epileptic syndromes associated 24–25, 28
subsyndromes 149
see also other specific entries

K
KCNQ1 gene 166
KCNQ2 gene 166, 181
KCNQ3 gene 161, 166, 181

L
Lafora's progressive myoclonus epilepsy 24,
146
age of onset 146
diagnosis 146
gene locus 146–149
tyrosine phosphatase gene mutation
148–149
lamotrigine 23, 114
Lennox–Gastaut syndrome
age of onset 135
frequency in first-degree relatives 138
genetics 133
linkage analysis 142, 175
childhood absence epilepsy and
chromosome 8q24 160–162
classic JME
chromosome 6p 151, 152
EJM1 gene (chromosome 6p21.3) 175,
176
idiopathic generalized epilepsy and
chromosome 15q14 190–194
JME with pyknoleptic absences and
chromosome 1p 154–156
multipoint 175, 176
localization-related epileptic activity in JME
38–39
LOD scores 199
chromosome 1p 155
chromosome 6p 151, 153, 163
chromosome 8q24 161, 162
chromosome 15q 183–184, 193
photogenic childhood absence with eyelid
myoclonia 157
long Q-T syndrome 166

M
magnetic resonance imaging (MRI) 22, 83
idiopathic generalized epilepsy 85–87
JME 85–87

quantitative studies 85–87
magnetoencephalography (MEG) 75, 76–77
case studies 78, 79
Marke–Nyman Inventory 104
maternal epilepsy 123, 125, 126
risk in children 132–133
medical disorders associated with JME
21–22
medical history 15
memory deficits 87, 105
mental disorders, in children after maternal
use of valproate 123
methsuximide 23
microdysgenesis 7, 94, 97
microsatellite markers 176, 177
middle-aged patients, JME 22
misdiagnosis 17–18, 24
JME stages causing 24–25
Molleret's triangle 57
motoneurons 57
motor evoked potentials (MEPs) 115
movement patterns 2
propulsive 7
retropulsive 7
murine jerky gene 165–166
myoclonic jerks 6, 13–14, 18
age at onset 16
case study 78
characteristics 18
corticospinal system activation 69
epilepsy relationship 6
frequency in JME 18, 20
incidence in absence epilepsies 136
photosensitivity and 48
preceding generalized tonic-clonic jerks 19
precipitation 115
response to antiepileptic drugs 114
spontaneous remission 114, 119
triggering factors 18
varying intensity 18
myoclonic status 18
myoclonus
EEG discharges relationship 61–63
pathophysiology *see* pathophysiology of
myoclonus

N
natural history of JME 22–23
neocortex
opioid release 93
structural changes 86, 87
neural tube defects 122
neuroimaging 22
neurological disorders, associated with JME
22
neuronal density, increased in JME 85, 86,
87

neurophysiology 106
  myoclonus 57–58
nicotinic acetylcholine receptor, neuronal
    177, 181–182
  α7 receptors 188
  functions 187
  genes 182
    susceptibility loci for JME 182–183
    see also CHRNA7 gene
  structure (representation) 186
  subunits 182, 185–186
    α7–α9 185–186
    structure (representation) 187
'noogenic epilepsies' 26
nucleus reticularis of thalamus, CHRNA7
    gene expression 187

O

offspring risks 130–131, 132, 141
olivo-dentato-rubro triangle 57
opiate receptors 93
opioids, release 93, 97
overtreatment 118
oxcarbazepine 24

P

parametric analysis 183, 192
paramyoclonus multiplex 6
partial motor seizures 38
pathology, of JME 83
pathophysiology of myoclonus 57–72
penetrance, definition 129
perioral myoclonias precipitated by talking
    and reading (PMPTR) 37
perioral reflex myoclonia 36, 37
personality changes 107
  in epilepsy 101, 102
personality disorders 21, 101
personality profile in JME 103–109, 107–108
  nonsubjective rating studies 103–104
petit mal, impulsive *see* impulsive petit mal
pharmacological sensitivity 24, 27
phenobarbital 23
phenytoin 23, 24
photogenic childhood absence with eyelid
    myoclonia 146, 159
  gene loci 146, 147, 156–157
photogenic epilepsy 26, 28
photoparoxysmal response 20, 47, 74
photosensitivity 19–20, 34, 74
  EEG findings 47–50, 74
  in JME 13, 19–20, 34, 48
  rate in relation to epilepsy types 48
positional cloning 174, 199
positron emission tomography (PET) 87
  applications 91
  idiopathic generalized epilepsy 91–99

isotopes used 91
potassium channel gene (KCNQ3) 161, 166,
    181
praxis 35, 37, 73
  precipitation in study 75
praxis-induced seizures 26, 35, 73–81, 199
  case studies 77–79
  evidence 73–81
  treatment and drug resistance 115
prefrontal cortex, dorsolateral 95
pregnancy 22
  valproate use during 121–128
prevalence, of JME 14, 83
primary reading epilepsy (PRE) 35–36
  JME combination 36–38
primidone 23
prognosis of JME 22–23, 27
  extratemporal structural changes 85
  relapse rate and 117
  without treatment 114
progressive familial myoclonus 6
progressive myoclonus, new syndrome
    24–25
progressive myoclonus epilepsy 24
properdin factor (Bf) 150
proprioceptive bombardment 38
psychiatric problems 20–21
puberty, prevalence of JME 13, 15
pyknoleptic absences 2
  in childhood absence epilepsy (CAE) 157
  in JME 150
    chromosome 1p locus 154–156
    gene loci associated 153–154
  types/patterns 2

R

reading epilepsy 35–36, 38
  secondary 36
recurrence risks, in offspring 130–131, 132,
    141
referral circumstances, JME 17
reflex epileptic traits 35, 38
reflex myoclonus 58
regional epileptic activity, in JME 38–39
relapse, in JME
  after drug discontinuation 111, 116–118,
    118–119
  rates 117
remission
  rates 112
  spontaneous 114, 119
reverse transcriptase polymerase chain
    reaction (RT-PCR) 188
Rolandic epilepsy 160

S

SADS rating scale 104

secondary psychomotor epilepsy, concept 106
secondary reading epilepsy 36
seizures
  cessation with antiepileptic therapy 113
  circadian distribution 20, 21
  circling 19
  combinations in JME 20
  cumulative incidence 129–130
  precipitation in JME 37
  as psychological regression 102
  recurrence during treatment 112–115
  relapse after treatment discontinuation
      116–118
  types in JME 13–14, 18–20, 27
    photosensitivity 13, 19–20, 34, 48, 76
    praxis-induced *see* praxis-induced
        seizures
  see also specific types of seizures
senile myoclonic epilepsy 25
sensory evoked potentials 75, 77, 79
severity of JME 22, 23
sex distribution 13, 15–16
sibling risks 131, 132, 133
single-stranded conformation polymorphism
    (SSCP) analysis, CHRNA7 gene 189
skull X-rays 84–85
sleep
  behaviour 102, 107
  effect on EEG 47
  profiles in JME 102–103
  REM 47
sleep deprivation 114
  effect on EEG in JME 47
sleep-wake cycle 7, 105–107
somatosensory evoked potentials 61
spina bifida aperta 121–122
spinal myoclonus 57
statistical parametric mapping (SPM) 94
stimuli, seizures influenced by 7
stress, seizures increase 23
structural changes in JME 83–89
sudden death, risks 23
susceptibility alleles 141–142
syndrome
  definition 33
  JME as xi, 33–39, 199

T
temporal lobe epilepsy 102
  personality profile comparisons 104

teratogenesis, maternal epilepsy and 126
teratogenicity, valproate 122, 126
thalamocortical system 69, 70, 92, 97
thalamus
  blood flow 92, 97
  CHRNA7 gene expression 187
  discharges starting in 87
tonic-clonic seizures on awakening, grey
    matter volume 85
topiramate 23
triggering factors, of JME 17, 19, 73, 105,
    112, 145
  avoidance 112, 116
  calculations and thinking 35
  myoclonic jerks 18
  nonspecific 112
  praxis *see* praxis
  reading 36, 37
  talking 37
    see also photosensitivity; praxis-induced
        seizures
twins
  concordance rates for idiopathic
      generalized epilepsy 137
  epilepsy 131
tyrosine phosphatase, gene mutation in
    Lafora's disease 148–149

U
underdiagnosis, of JME 11
Unverricht-Lundborg epilepsy 24

V
valproate 23, 121
  dosages in pregnancy 122, 125
  effect on flumazenil binding 94, 95–96
  low-dose 22
  maternal use during pregnancy 121–128
  response in JME 111, 112, 113, 115
  seizure recurrence during treatment
      113
visual stimuli 19
Vitamin Study Research Group of MRC
    126

W
Wechsler Intelligence Scale 104, 123
West syndrome 2, 7, 138
  genetics 133
Wisconsin Card Sorting test 105